DIVINE APPOINTMENT

My Red Rover Team, brothers Jimmy and Billy

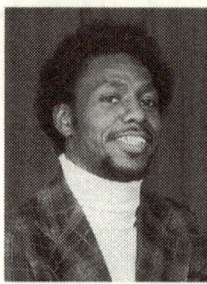

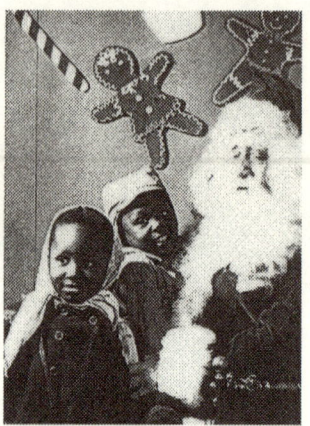

My brother, William
"Billy" Lewis (deceased)

Little boy with stupid grin, James (Jimmy)
Lewis; cute little girl, Delores (Cookie)
Thornton; fat white man, Santa (not on the
team: O). Taken in 1954.

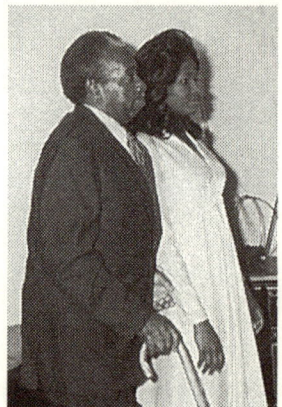

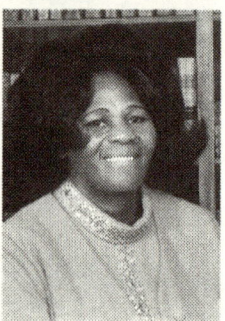

My mom, Daisy Lewis

My dad, Chester Lewis
(deceased), and me, 1976

DIVINE APPOINTMENT

A Caregiver's Guide

Delores Thornton

iUniverse, Inc.
New York Lincoln Shanghai

Divine Appointment
A Caregiver's Guide

iUniverse, Inc.

For information address:
iUniverse, Inc.
2021 Pine Lake Road, Suite 100
Lincoln, NE 68512
www.iuniverse.com

Information obtained from research came from "Communicate to Stay Healthy: Talk to Your Pharmacist" and is used with permission of the Indiana Pharmacy Alliance. The "Most Frequently Asked Questions" section is reprinted from, Caregiving Tips Most FAQ, with permission of the National Family Caregivers Association, Kensington, MD, the nation's only organization for all family caregivers. 1-800-986-3650; www.nfcacares.org.
This book contains a few words from various caregivers. They are credited at the beginning of the chapters in which their work is found. This book also contains two poems by unknown authors. All other work is that of the author, including short-short stories, anecdotes and poems.
Scripture taken from the HOLY BIBLE, NEW INTERNATIONAL VERSION®. Copyright 1973, 1978, 1984 by International Bible Society. Used by permission of Zondervan. All rights reserved.
LCCN: 2004093032

ISBN: 0-595-31897-5

Printed in the United States of America

I dedicate this work to Caregivers everywhere. God Bless You All!

"Let All Things Be Done Decently And In Order"

I Corinthians 14:40

CONTENTS

▼

Preface

Divine Appointment: A Caregiver's Guide is my personal story. It contains short-short stories and anecdotes as well as legal, medical, and psychological information. I spent countless hours interviewing caregivers, and although I don't know all that there is to know about the subject, what I do know I freely share. I was thrust into a caregiver's world in which I knew nothing, and I had to learn quickly. I prayed to God for answers, and his replies are contained in this guide. Through the grace of The Holy Spirit I was allowed to pen this work to act as an aid and inspiration for others who find themselves looking forward to a brighter tomorrow, or even those who are "walking through the valley of the shadow of death!" In all probability most of us will become caregivers at some point in our lives.

It is important for us to realize that dying is a necessary part of living. If we make preparations it will lessen the burdens of our loved ones. I did extensive research and spoke with newspaper and magazine editors, funeral home directors, and cemetery personnel to glean as much information on this topic as I possibly could. I pray that *Divine Appointment: A Caregiver's Guide* will be useful to you and your loved ones. God Bless!

Foreword

Too many of us want to escape from thoughts of our loved ones falling victim to illness, and we rarely stop to seriously consider how we would care for them if the worst scenario presented itself. Nevertheless, life and death, and sickness and health are polar opposites that eventually meet and fuse. Tomorrow is not promised to any of us, despite age, sex, race, or income level. At any given moment someone can lose the ability to care for him or herself. Then what must a loved one do? How will the person closest to the infirm cope? More importantly, how will he or she react? Decisions must be made, and there is not much time to make them.

Someone in the patient's life must quickly step up to the plate, gather his or her faculties, and begin preparing for life following a loved one's diagnosis. The daughter, son, wife, mother, father, husband, or significant other suddenly becomes more than someone who shares bloodlines or a wedding vow. At this point that person becomes a caregiver and must carry a heavy burden. The weight of the burden is twofold: One part involves the emotional difficulty of watching a loved one suffer, and the other is the added responsibility of meeting the constant need of someone who needs you for small and great things alike.

Most people thrust into this situation are without medical training and are unprepared for the journey they are about to take. What will the road toward becoming a caregiver be like? What types of issues should be addressed? It is easy to understand the incredible sense of responsibility and confusion that may threaten to swallow a person in this position whole.

But what if such a person could pick up a book and read helpful information that would inform, guide, and comfort? Delores Thornton's *Divine Appointment: A Caregiver's Guide* bridges this gap by addressing an often unrecognized segment of the population. For this reason her work is an indispensable reference tool that should be a part of every professional and home library. Thornton has given us a priceless gift in the form of a book that is devoted to examining the full breadth of dilemmas which a caregiver, and the person who is cared for, endure when illness sets in and the possibility of a loved one's death looms near. What she observed, felt, and experienced as a caregiver will shed light upon what it is like to be in this position. Having this information at a caregiver's disposal will lessen his or her burden of feeling overwhelmed and will instruct them how to start putting things in order and organizing them into manageable tasks.

The author's loving spirit leaps off the pages, and I doubt that anyone will turn the last page of her book not feeling more equipped to handle a tough situation with grace. As the author recounts her personal experiences, you will be informed on how to cope, and you will be encouraged to lean on God to make it through your storm. You will even understand the many facets of what a caregiver you know may be going through. Receive Delores Thornton's words with gratefulness, for she was inspired to share her touching story with you. Welcome to one of the most important literary journeys that you will ever take…welcome to the world of a caregiver.

Andrea Blackstone

Acknowledgments

I thank God for giving me the vision for this work!

I'd also like to thank the following:

Joe for being so kind, even when you were confused or in intense pain.

My family for giving me moral support.

Lena, my dear friend and also president of the Friendgurlz Book Club. You've always been here for me, and I owe you soooo much.

Bob Coalson who has worked with me on every project I've undertaken. Your professionalism seems to shine through every book I write.

Cynthia Whisler, Managing Funeral Director at Crown Hill Funeral Home and Cemetery. The phone interviews and the taped sessions really proved to be invaluable as I worked to flesh out all of the information you gave. God Bless You!

Michelle Neimier for supplying me with invaluable information about facilities for patients and other resources for caregivers.

Vanessa Johnson, a new friend whom I met online. I asked her to share some of her experiences in dealing with grief and loss. I presented questions like: I'd like to know how your mom and son died since you said they were untimely. I'd also like to know how you dealt with it. Did you experience anger? Guilt? How rough was your road to recovery? What got you *through*? How are you doing now? I've included her story in chapter 13. Additionally, I thank Vanessa for the list of websites on grief and loss.

And Other Caregivers:

> Kenya Carr for bearing her soul, although it was painful! I know that heaven is pleased with you.

Janet Lewis who provided information about Agnes (her mother), who suffered a stroke in the early 1990s.

Barbara Custer, author of *Twilight Healer*, who writes the following:
"I'm a caregiver myself. Mike (my husband) has tremor-predominant Parkinson's Disease. That means that tremor is the dominant symptom, while the other symptoms are mild. Mike's tremor got so bad, though, that he couldn't hold a cup of water.

He wasn't able to tolerate the medicines to contain his symptoms, so he had a procedure done called deep brain stimulation (implants in the brain). This has controlled his tremor nicely; however, he has developed other medical problems which further compromise his independence. Mike also has Osteoarthritis, and it so bad in his right knee that he can hardly walk."

To all of the instructors and students of Simmons Bible College, I say thanks so much for helping me to grow.
I'd also like to thank some of my online friends:

AALBC/Troy Johnson

Anutwistaflava/ Monique Baldwin

African-American Lit.

APOOO/Yasmin Coleman

SORMAG/LaShaunda Hoffman

BWunited/Tia Shabazz

Book-Remarks/Cyndey Rax

Booksigners Authors/Moderator Shirley Dicks

Authors For Charity/Shirley Dicks

Black Expression 2004 Group/Sachel

Disilgold/Heather Covington

C&B Books Distribution/Carol Rogers & Brenda Piper

DOENETWORK/Tyora Moody

SistaGirl Book Club/Kenyatta Ingram

RAWSISTAZ/Tee C. Royal

The RealReviewers/Jacki Miller

The Writers' Crib

ITCOMS (In the Company of My Sistah's Book Club) The President of ITCOMS is Victoria Jourdan

MWC/Gloria Anglón

Nubian Sistas Book Club/Joy Farrington

Readincolor Book Club/Angie Pickett-Henderson

TNC/Shonell Bacon

Sexy Ebony BBW African American Book Club/Founder, Dee-Dee AKA DD

Writing Warriors For Christ

OneSwan Productions/Janette Owens

BlackRefer.com/Woodie

Good Book Club/Pamela Walker Williams

Authors Helping Authors/Andrea Blackstone

To all of the members of my two Internet Groups:

Marguerite Press Promo

Marguerite Press

Finally, I thank all of the bookstores, reading groups, librarians, newspapers, magazines, and book clubs for your support of this book.

Chapter 1

▼

Bio of a Caregiver

One of the most rewarding forms of missionary work is the church missionary, which is often a lifelong calling. Missionaries are responsible for spreading the word about the joy of being a Christian and for converting others. Some people put missionaries on the same level as evangelists and apostles. As a small child growing up in Indianapolis my mother sent me and my six older siblings to worship at the Church of the Nazarene. By age nine I was singing in the choir and fellowshiping at a church in Haughville called Second Timothy Baptist.

My mother had 11 children at the time and rarely accompanied us to church, but she held Bible drills every Wednesday, which reinforced everything that we'd learned at Sunday School and Prayer Meeting. One day while out playing I saw a beautiful sign in the church yard of First Baptist Church (located around the corner from me) announcing an upcoming summer session for Bible school. I desired more information so I went inside, signed up, and promised the teachers that I'd return with more neighborhood children. It wasn't an easy task to convince playmates to leave hopscotch, jump ropes, and dolls behind, but I accomplished it! The nightly events of Vacation Bible School included arts, crafts, Bible verses, and singing. I think most of my friends attended because of the ham sandwiches and cookies that were served at the end of each night. But I received total joy hearing the stories about Jesus. There were also puzzles of Noah, Samson, Jonah, Ruth, and other Bible greats.

When Vacation Bible School concluded I felt a great loss. No longer would I go through the side door of First Baptist where the picture of Jesus greeted all visitors, members, and friends. At age 11 my family and I moved to another part of town, and I never visited my former church again. I can't recall the Church Mother's name, but I still see her soft angelic face. I still hear her saying, " Chile, you gonna be a missionary."

Through the years I've been in and out of church, but I've never felt that I was out of touch with God. I've worked on different committees and auxiliaries—pastor's aid, nurses, ushers, and various choirs. Additionally, I've organized fundraisers and given programs to aid the church.

In 2002, I was led by the Holy Spirit to educate and prepare myself for my missionary ministry. To that end I enrolled in classes at Simmons Bible College, Indianapolis Extension. Under the tutelage of the likes of Reverend Joseph Wilkins, Reverend Charles Ellis, Jr., Reverend L. Wayne Smith, and Olivia Gonzales, I've had a wealth of knowledge at my disposal. I now feel qualified to join the Missionary Society of my church (Greater St. Mark, MBC). I am now ready to heed my purpose and answer my calling which is to draw souls to Jesus, who is the joy of my life.

Things to Think About

It is a wonderful thing to care about people and what happens to them! In the 1980s my mother-in-law was diagnosed with terminal cancer. She immediately made her funeral arrangements and even gave the family a strange request. She didn't want a funeral procession to follow her to the cemetery for she'd had a nightmare in which we were all leaving the cemetery, and she could see us but couldn't get up to come with us. I thought about that in 2003, when I noticed an eerie sight!

Death Unnoticed

It was a sad sight to see the hearse driving down Kessler Blvd. The top was laden with flowers. There were the floral sprays that usually adorn a casket, arrangements of spring flowers being washed by torrential rains, and even smaller flowers in urns.

There was no car of pall bearers,
No flowers girls,
No family cars carrying bereaved loved ones.

Who eulogized?
Who sympathized?
Who announced that dinner would be served at the church?
Who sang a song?
Who played along?
Who spoke of the decedent's worth?

There were no ushers with fans to pass out,
No shouting or fainting that we heard about.

Only a hearse going down Kessler Blvd.,
That turned slowly and entered the gate;
There were no cries
From passersby,
Not even an escort to make folks wait!

Scripture Reference:

Train up a child in the way he should go: and when he is old, he will not depart from it.

Proverbs 22:6

CHAPTER 2

▼

STORM WARNING

Most illnesses don't come on suddenly, but rather they advance through certain stages. Just as tornadoes and other storms give notice of imminent danger, so too does the body. It is for this reason that it is wise to recognize early warning signs. Doctors have suggested that it is not wise to take over-the-counter medicines or use home remedies to mask pain. Pain is a signal that something somewhere is out-of-balance. A simple headache could mean potential eye problems; dizziness could signal hypertension; constant thirst could mean onset of diabetes.

It is extremely important to maintain a healthy life-style, complete with diet and exercise. I became a primary caregiver in October of 2003. My fiancé (Joe) had passed out in a local supermarket. Paramedics were called, and he was taken to a local hospital here in Indianapolis. He remained in the "Emergency Room" for several hours while doctors ran extensive tests. Joe didn't have a primary care physician, so upon his discharge he was advised to return to the hospital for follow-up visits.

It wasn't until about September that his newly-appointed doctor informed him that he had indeed suffered a mild stroke. This sounded so strange to Joe and me, for we had always assumed that heart attacks and strokes were easily recognized. We didn't realize that sometimes evidence of stroke doesn't appear until months down the line. Although doctors treat the stroke symptoms, they don't classify the condition as stroke until conclusive data is in.

There were endless doctor's visits and numerous trips to the outpatient services in the hospital. This was an experience in and of itself. Strolling the corridors of a massive hospital wasn't made easier by the maps at the information desk. Upon arriving at the destination, I was surprised to see the signs that read "Point to your language and wait for a translator."

Services Available:
  French
  Arabic
  Japanese
  German
  Thai
  Vietnamese
  Korean
  Spanish

I suppose this is a sign of the times. On this particular visit Joe was having an "Echo Stress Test," which is a heart test. He was ushered into an examining room and told to undress. Cold cream was then applied to his upper body, and a monitor was strapped around his waist for the heart ultrasound. The purpose was to look for changes in the walls of the heart. Next Joe was asked to get on the treadmill, and he immediately informed the technician that he felt as though he were falling backwards. One of the technicians instructed him to move forward nearer the handle bars. After he completed the treadmill, he had to sit on the side of the bed and remain perfectly still for two minutes. Then the technicians administered the heart ultrasound a second time. After approximately one hour the test was complete, and we were on our way home.

The next day we visited the primary care physician who told him to give up smoking and drinking. I was ecstatic, but the withdrawal caused Joe extreme anxiety.

Things to Think About

Storms will enter our lives, and not all will give advance warnings. Sometimes we get a feeling that conditions are favorable for certain storms.

Scripture Reference:
Acts 27:27-31

But when the fourteenth night was come, as we were driven up and down in Adria, about midnight the shipmen deemed that they drew near to some country; And sounded, and founded it twenty fathoms: and when they had gone a little further, they sounded again, and found fifteen fathoms. Then fearing lest we should have fallen upon rocks, they cast four anchors out of the stern, and wished for the day. And as the shipmen were about to flee out of the ship, when they had let down the boat into the sea, under colour as though they would have cast anchors out of the foreship, Paul said to the centurion and to the soldiers, Except these abide in the ship, ye cannot be saved.

CHAPTER 3

▼

RED ROVER

As a child growing up I was sandwiched in between two brothers, one two years my senior and the other two years my junior. Since I didn't have any sisters near my own age, I became a tomboy. Always short and small, I didn't fare very well when it came time to being placed on teams for sports. I couldn't outrun the boys, couldn't out-bat them, and certainly couldn't kick as far. Somehow though I remember always getting in the game, if but for only a short while.

One of my favorite games was "Red Rover." In that game all of the members of one team clasped their hands around each others' wrists, to form a human chain. It was the job of the opposing team to crash through the line after hearing, "Red Rover, Red Rover, we dare one of you over!" For some reason (that I later figured out) all of the opponents came straight at me. More often than not they broke through, but not always. My older brother suggested to our teammates that our two strongest players stand on either side of me. From then on the opposing players sought to find another weak link, for I had been strengthened.

A lot of lonely sleepless nights when Joe was depressed or having adverse reactions to medicines, I thought of Red Rover. When Joe demanded a gun to protect himself from the red people, I comforted and reassured him, telling him it was just another hallucination. I realized that the enemy was seeking to break through in areas he presumed to be weak. During those times I tried to stay prayed up. I drew so close to my strength that there was no way for the enemy to gain the victory.

Things to think about

The enemy will always attack in vulnerable places, so it's wise to hold onto God's Unchanging Hand. When the enemy yells, "Red Rover," The Lord won't forsake you, and won't let you go!

Scripture Reference:
Matthew 9:37, 38

> Then saith he to his disciples, The harvest truly is plenteous, but the laborers are few. Pray ye therefore the Lord of the harvest, that he will send forth laborers into his harvest.

CHAPTER 4

▼

ELBOW GREASE

When I was eleven years old my parents moved my eleven siblings and myself to a new home. My father was a strong family man who worked tirelessly to feed and clothe his brood. When we moved from the two bedroom home to a large spacious house on the north side of Indianapolis, he was quite proud. He called the new home his "castle," and as such he was determined to keep it immaculate. One of the things he did was instruct his children on how to scrub and shine the railings and banisters.

One day while my Uncle Sonny was visiting, I decided to impress him by singing *Sweeping Through the City,* an old Negro spiritual made famous by the Caravans. Uncle Sonny had been a member of various gospel singing groups, and I loved his deep baritone voice. Daddy came into the room just as I was breaking into the chorus and shouted that I shouldn't be sweeping, I should be washing the banisters. Dipping the Pinesol-soaked rag into the cold water, I rubbed it softly across the surface, still hoping that Uncle Sonny was enjoying my song. Daddy looked at the area I was cleaning then shook his head. "You need to put some elbow grease on that!" he said loudly.

I looked at Uncle Sonny and winked. "We don't have anymore elbow grease," I replied. All of us knew that whenever we played dumb, it really made Daddy mad.

"I swear, the older y'all get, the dumber y'all get," he said as he went out to the front yard to dig in his flowers.

I always knew that applying elbow grease meant to dig deep, but I never realized just how hard it would be and how much elbow grease I would need to get through situations in my adult life. But I found out in the fall of 2003!

*   *   *   *

Just when we thought things were getting back to normal, the unthinkable happened. I was upstairs on the computer checking email messages when Joe hollered up and announced that he was going to bed. My teenage granddaughter, who was spending the weekend, had just settled down to watch music videos on BET. It was 11 p.m. when I logged off of the Internet and prepared for bed. I showered, said my prayers, and was in bed by 11:30 p.m. I picked up the remote control from my pillow and turned to CNN. Joe turned to face me and I figured I had awakened him. I asked if the television was bothering him—he just stared at me, and didn't answer. Lying there in the dark with the only light illuminating from the television screen, it seemed as though Joe was angry. He stared wildly at me. Sometimes the different medicines made him extremely irritable. I turned the television off and rolled over to face the wall. Almost immediately the bed started to shake as if we were in the middle of an earthquake registering a five on the Richter Scale.

I sprang from the bed and turned on the light. Joe was trembling and making loud gurgling sounds! I ran to the kitchen, snatched up the cordless phone, and dialed 911. "Stay on the line," the dispatcher instructed after I told her there was a possible stroke victim. I started to the closet to get dressed, but the dispatcher told me to stay right at the bedside. I was instructed to roll Joe over on his side and remove the pillows.

After what seemed like a small eternity, the paramedics arrived. I threw on a robe and let them in. Meanwhile I'd asked my frightened granddaughter to call one of my daughters to come and drive us to the hospital, for I was entirely too nervous. Three of the paramedics worked on Joe while the fourth one took me into the kitchen to give him the personal information necessary for the admitting desk. I was so upset I couldn't even remember Joe's birth date. By the time I found the social security card and other pertinent information, they were rolling Joe out the front door. When I asked about his condition they informed me that it didn't look good.

Within minutes my daughter arrived. I threw on a T-shirt and a pair of jeans, then slipped on a pair of mules. This time Joe wasn't released after a few hours. He'd suffered a massive stroke and a seizure. The doctors asked me about a living will, and also about coding him. I was at a loss again! Since I was only his fianceé, I couldn't sign any papers for treatment. And, I couldn't even remember any of his three daughters' phone numbers.

Things to think about

Try to have all important information in a handy place. It would be nice to have this for all family members including children who no longer live at home. Discuss loved ones' preferences while they're well; then you can abide by their wishes. If you are not related, you might try to get power of attorney when you become a caregiver. If a Living Will has been drawn up, it will make matters easier for all concerned. This is a declaration that is recognized as a legal document in most of the United States. In it the person states the measures that the medical profession should or should not take to sustain life. It states the person's legal right to refuse treatments that might prolong life and even deals with resuscitation, artificial feeding, and artificial respiration.

Additionally, the person may give specific instructions on procedures and practices to be done for them. Doctors are bound by this and are held blameless and free from legal ramifications. In the Living Will Declaration the person may also designate another to act on their behalf should they become incapacitated. The Living Will Declaration must be signed and dated and must also be witnessed by two people.

Since the Living Will is a constitutional right, most hospitals will ask if you have one upon admittance. It is suggested that people make several copies of their Living Will. Keep the original with other important documents at home; give copies to close family members, attorneys, and physicians. As with your regular will, you may want to review and revise your Living Will from time to time. When this happens make certain that you share your change of mind with the persons to whom you've given copies of your Living Will.

Preparing A Will

Although it is possible to make a will without an attorney, it is strongly recommended that one be consulted. There are complex issues that the survivors and executors will encounter if the testator (one making the will) has not written the will correctly.

Things to consider when planning your will:

- It would be wise to develop several options in the event that your first choice of beneficiary predeceases you.
- List two executors in the event that one is either unable or unwilling to carry out the duties contained in your will.
- If married you should include your spouse's full name, address, social security number, date of marriage
- Names and birth dates of all children (date of death if applicable)
- Any children with disabilities?
- Names of children from previous marriages
- List grandchildren and anything which you'd like for them to inherit
- At what age would you like for your children to be able to manage their inheritance?
- Are you or your spouse Legal Guardians of any minors?
- Are there previous spouses?
- Make sure that you designate the family and friends who you'd like to inherit family heirlooms. Many times this is a cause of squabbles among survivors!
- List all of your debts
- List all assets, including: real estate, jewelry, cars, bank accounts, tools, household items, life insurance policies, antiques, savings bonds, stamp collections and some retirement plans.
- Do you have an safety deposit boxes? List the location and box number. Who has access?

Definition of terms:

- Testator—person making the Will
- Executor—person appointed to carry out the terms of the Will
- Guardian—a person with legal rights to act in the best interests of persons who are unable to take care of themselves.
- Beneficiary—one who is named by the testator in the Will, to receive money and/or property.

The list above contains basic information which might help your attorney as you prepare your will.

Some thoughts on Euthanasia

Euthanasia has always been a difficult topic for me to come to terms with. Since childhood I've seen the cowboy shoot the wounded horse, and it aroused no concern for I felt it was the best thing to do. To put an animal out of misery seems a simple solution. However, when dealing with humans there are nagging questions. The controversy encompasses the right to die issues. In this chapter I offer some of the things I've discovered through my research on the topic of euthanasia.

Although life expectancy rates have risen steadily since the 1940s, the quality of life for senior citizens has been a cause for concern. Some elderly patients with terminal illnesses bring financial burdens on their families and also present a strain on the community at large. For these reasons there are currently pleas for legislation that will legalize certain types of euthanasia.

The arguments over euthanasia go back to the ancient world. The Stoics favored it while the Pythagoreans were against it. Even Plato approved it in some cases of terminal illness. Although for the most part Greeks favored euthanasia, Hippocrates (the ancient Greek physician) was strongly opposed. His oath states emphatically that life should be preserved, and it also asserts that the good of patients must be placed above the interests of the physician. The *Hippocratic Oath* is still taken by doctors today before they enter their various fields of practice.

When patients are in a vegetative state and have not made a living will nor designated a power of attorney, others have painful decisions to make on their behalf. If there have been no arrangements for the care, then family members must make decisions concerning when to end life-sustaining measures. Permission to end life-sustaining measures to terminal patients is quite different from assisted suicide.

While discussing euthanasia, there are various relevant concepts to present. Voluntary euthanasia takes place when the patient gives consent in either a verbal or written statement (a living will). Voluntary euthanasia is sometimes equated with suicide. Involuntary euthanasia is when the patient is unconscious or comatose and unable to give consent. In these cases it is typically a member of the family who makes the decision. This would surely be considered murder by many people.

There are additional terms referred to when discussing euthanasia: *direct* euthanasia is when the patient makes the decision to die, *indirect* euthanasia is when another party acts out the decision. *Death with dignity* deals with allowing patients to die a natural death—that is, without living solely through the aid of machines. When the terminally-ill patient is allowed to die under these circumstances, it is not normally considered suicide. *Mercy killing* is defined as the releasing of a patient who is in excruciating pain, and there is nothing to control it. Some cancer patients fall into this category when morphine is no longer effective, and they experience what doctors call break-away pain. Mercy killing at the request of the patient is also considered suicide. *Death selection* is the removal of persons whose lives are no longer considered socially useful. People should be careful of this idea, for it is an extremely dangerous social concept, as persons involved might not even be ill, but perhaps criminals, misfits, or considered as in some way undesirable.

Utilitarian views support euthanasia. Utilitarian decisions on who lives or dies could possibly be based on who is thought to be most beneficial to society. *Deontological* (moral theories according to the rightness or obligatoriness of an action is not exclusively determined by the value of its consequences) views are considered non-utilitarian.

The Christian perspective speaks to an afterlife and suggests that death is a part of life, a gift from God. Scripture is clearly against suicide, be it voluntary/involuntary, passive/active, killing or letting die. Christians to whom I have spoken feel that since God gives life and sustains it, it is to be cherished and considered sacred. They further note that there is much to learn through suffering. Since persons are made in God's own image, to take that life is sin! God is still in the miracle business, so no one has a right to actively participate in or passively allow euthanasia.

I come from a very large family, and there is a prevalence of cancer and other agonizing diseases. I have seen loved ones lose their minds, their eyesight, and even their will to live. I've heard them cry out in excruciating pain.

My feelings about euthanasia and/or mercy killings springs from all of the pain I've witnessed. I have always felt that terminally-ill patients in severe pain should have the right to decide whether to live or die. But now I am forced to re-think my position, which has been morally incorrect. I now realize that all life is precious and, as such, should be preserved. I have come to the conclusion that death is a necessary part of life, and we all have an appointed time to die! But while you are yet alive, you will have to give life your all, using the elbow grease.

Scriptural Reference:

A fool despiseth his father's instruction: be he that regarded reproof is prudent.

Proverbs 15:5

CHAPTER 5

▼

BALD BLONDE

In the mid-nineties, I connected with a woman through my literary pursuits. As a matter of fact, she called my business number to say that she had read my debut novel, *Ida Mae*. We started talking and since she was in the newspaper business, she offered to help me get the word out about my literary entrepreneurship. We talked on the phone for several months, and she even wrote an article about me in her senior citizens' publication. One day she called and said she wanted to meet me, so we arranged a lunch at an area restaurant.

Before hanging up the phone I realized that we didn't have descriptions of each other, so I told her that I was a middle-age black woman. I gave her the make and model of my car in the event that we pulled up at the same time. After holding the line for a moment, she replied, "Oh, I won't be hard to spot; I'm a bald blonde."

I was tempted to laugh, but something told me not to. Instead I told her that I'd see her the following Tuesday at the appointed time. When Tuesday rolled around, I pulled up on the lot of the restaurant and looked for my phone-friend's car. I didn't see it, so I went inside the restaurant. I asked the hostess if anyone had come in looking for a Delores Thornton.

"Sure, your party is right over there," the hostess said, pointing cheerfully.

"Thank you," I replied as I edged closer to the table where my friend sat. She stood and shook my hand, smiling warmly as she did.

"I'm so glad to finally meet you," she said.

"Yes, I feel the same way," I answered.

We ordered lunch, and in between bites we chatted like old friends. I couldn't help but notice that not only was she bald, but she had no eyebrows or eyelashes. Other than those disturbing flaws, she was a very attractive lady. I wondered if she'd had chemotherapy, but she didn't volunteer any information, and I didn't pry. When the lunch was over, we started toward the cashier.

"Hand me your bill," she said. "This one's on me."

"You really don't have to," I replied as I put the bill in her milky-white hand. Although she may have been suffering from alopecia (a scalp condition), I was convinced that she was a cancer patient, more importantly a cancer survivor.

"I know," she replied, "but the next time it's on you."

We exchanged goodbyes and promised to stay in touch, but we didn't. All the way to the car I wondered about my phone friend. Why did she call herself a bald blonde. And then it hit me, it is not what others think of you, but what you think of yourself! Sometimes when we look at people, we only see the outside, but there is so much more to learn if people will only peel away the superficial elements of life.

I wondered how Joe saw himself. Surely he complained about having to walk so slowly, but it wasn't just his walk. His reaction time was slowed, his speech slurred, and he began to talk louder. Always in a state of depression, his appetite waned, and he lost weight. He started to feel better after going to a few of the outpatient therapy sessions. One such clinic gave him oral pharyngeal exercises to help with his swallowing. During those visits he did 10 to 15 repetitions of the following exercises: lips, tongue, tongue base, hyolaryngeal elevation, laryngeal elevation, pharyngeal wall movement, and swallowing maneuvers.

Joe had a condition called *Dysphagia*, something I'd never heard of. To think that something as instinctive as swallowing would be lost to stroke patients was a bit hard for me to grasp. The doctors informed us that Joe was not swallowing properly, and he had to add a thickener to all liquids and go on a water (Frasier) protocol. This meant that he couldn't drink water within 30 minutes of eating, and then only after he'd brushed his teeth and removed all food particles from his mouth.

One of the things that really amazed me was the thickener which Joe had to use to add to all liquids. We were told that since his swallow was not right, food could be washed down into his lungs with liquids. It was so foreign to think of someone who couldn't swallow, but that is what happens with some stroke victims. Due to the damage of the brain, the patient has to go through therapy to retrain the muscles that allow swallowing. In the event that liquids enter the lungs, pneumonia becomes a concern. Since the lungs can tolerate water, that is the only thing that certain stroke victims can drink without adding a thickener. At times when Joe wanted to attend social functions or funerals, we had to pack applesauce or liquids along with the thickener which was placed in sandwich bags. He used the thickened liquids and/or applesauce to swallow his pills.

At first Joe had to be on a honey liquid consistency, then he graduated to nectar thick. He had to limit his intake to single sips of liquid, and was told to sit up straight during meals and to sit upright for 30 minutes following each meal. Once a month he had to visit the outpatient department of the hospital to have a swallow study done. At that time technicians would give him liquids then monitor him to see if his swallow had improved. Finally after three long months he passed the swallow study! He was able to drink regular liquids and no longer had to follow the Frazier protocol.

Although most of his physical therapy involved arm exercises with five pound weights, there were also leg exercises which he did daily. It was also suggested that he start walking regularly, and he reluctantly complied.

Another area we had to work on was his consumption of sodium. We started studying labels at the supermarket and found that most foods were extremely high in sodium. Frozen and canned foods were the biggest enemies. Shopping for low sodium meals was quite exhausting, and all of our favorite foods were out. The doctor advised Joe to stay below 2,000 mg. of sodium per day. There were spices and seasonings that had to be abandoned. But we were pleasantly surprised to find Morton salt substitute. It tasted even better than salt!

Things to think about:
Adopting a Healthy Lifestyle

It would be wise for all people to practice healthy habits early in life and reduce their risk of heart attack and stroke in later years. To do this start looking at labels now.

Scriptural Reference:

And a certain man was there which had an infirmity thirty and eight years. When Jesus saw him lie, and knew that he had been now a long time in that case, he saith unto him, 'Wilt thou be made whole?' The impotent man answered him, 'Sir, I have no man, when the water is troubled, to put me into the pool; but while I am coming another steppeth down before me.' Jesus saith unto him, 'Rise, take up thy bed, and walk.'

John 5:5-8

CHAPTER 6

▼

THE MEDICINE CABINET

When I was a young child, back in the *olden days* (as my children refer to my youth), my siblings and I would have to endure some of the worse medicines known to man. For illnesses there was goose grease, Father John, Cod Liver Oil, Caster Oil, and sautéed onions with a flour mixture. Those were the cure-all's for whatever ailed you. Of course the nasty dosages were usually washed down with a big juicy orange, but sometimes the medicines even made the oranges taste bitter. My parents assured us that because the medicines were so disgusting, they were doing a good job of making us better. That might have been true in the olden days, but due to advances in modern medicine, more agents and chemicals are being used. For that reason it is imperative that people check the dates on medicines and not use them past the expiration date. Just because the medicines have a nasty taste or foul odor doesn't mean that they're good for you!

Trying to keep up with all of the medicines can prove to be a monumental task. There were times when Joe was about to run out of medicine, and I had to call the doctor's office to have them phone in a refill to our neighborhood pharmacy. Trying to keep up with seven or eight medicines became taxing, as when I noticed that one prescription was low and got a refill, and there would be two or three others that were just as close to the bottom of the bottle. Some of the pills were once a day, others twice a day, and still others three times a day. Then there was the Catapress patch for high blood pressure which Joe had to wear everyday. The patch had to be changed once a week.

Since the costs of the medicines were so high, at times we attempted to get half of them filled. That turned out to be a mistake, for when I went back to the pharmacy to get the other half, they said there were no more refills. When I called the doctor's office, they told me it was an error on the part of the pharmacy. The constant mix-up of the prescriptions was a headache in and of itself.

A few of the medicines, or perhaps the combination of all of them, caused nightmares and hallucinations. There were times when Joe would awake in the middle of the night trembling. He'd seen snakes and ghosts, heard knocking at the front door. He even saw a "red woman" who commanded him to get up from the couch as he was watching television. He even demanded that I return his gun to him which I had put away for fear that he would shoot me or, even worse, one of my grown children who come by to visit. When he wasn't having nightmares, he was waking me up to argue; those days were truly a test for me. I know that a weaker person would have reacted differently, but I had to remind myself that this person wasn't really Joe.

The doctor's visits were just as complex as the regimen of medicines. Once when Joe had a bad reaction to a medicine, his doctor told me to bring him into the office the next day. When we arrived, the receptionist informed us that Joe didn't have an appointment. After about 15 minutes the problem was resolved, and we went in to see the doctor. Joe had developed another condition, a side effect of one of the medicines he was taking. He was referred to a specialist. I couldn't believe it when I took him to the specialist that next week: The doctor kept him in the examining room for only five minutes! He said we'd have to reschedule for he didn't have the reports from the referring physician. So that was a wasted trip!

Things to Think About:
Keeping Up with the Medicines

Make a list and keep it with you, and also give the patient a copy. Post a copy of the list on the refrigerator. Check off the medicines daily until you establish a habit of administering them. You might also purchase a pill box and place all of the doses for the day in it. Then it will be easy to determine if a dosage has been missed. This may seem like a small thing, but with all of the stress of caring for the patient, sometimes things will slip by you. Improper medication can advance disease and even cause death. It is also good to understand that the worse place for medicine is in the medicine cabinet in the bathroom since this room has high humidity. Some people are also under the false impression that storing medicine in the refrigerator is a good thing. But it is unwise to store medicines there unless the pharmacist label on the bottle says to do so.

Proper Use of Medications

Studies show that 50% of all medications are taken incorrectly.
Why are medications taken improperly?

- Patients think the medication is unnecessary or not working.

- Patients feel better and stop taking their medication.

- Medication side effects.

- Doses are forgotten or inconvenient to take.

- Directions are misunderstood due to language barriers or illiteracy.

Understand the answers to these questions from your physician or pharmacist.

- What is the name of my medication?

- Why am I taking it?

- When and how do I take it?

- How long is the medication therapy? Short term or long term?

- What side effects could I expect? What should I do if they happen?

- What should I do if I miss a dose?

- Are there any special storage conditions?

Pharmacists can help you understand your medications.

- Try to have all your prescriptions filled at the same pharmacy (or chain) to keep your medication record up to date. If you go to a different pharmacy, give them a list of medications you take (prescription and non-prescription).

- Keep a list with you of all the medications you take. List any allergies and medical conditions on this paper.

- Tell your pharmacist when your medications change so your profile can be kept current.

- Ask your pharmacist about non-prescription medications, vitamins, and herbal products. Your pharmacist can help you choose a medication that will not interact with your other medications. He may also suggest generic drugs that tend to cost less.

- Use reminders to help you remember to take your medications (medication boxes). Make a schedule and keep to it.

- For help with costs, check these drug assistance programs.

  - www.helpingpatients.org

  - www.freemedicine.com

  - www.benefitscheckuprx.com

- Use reliable Internet sources for information.

Check your medicine chest, and make sure you have the following items:

Thermometer for all household members

A blood pressure cuff

An easy-acting laxative

Regular Tylenol (a lot of patients can't take aspirin)

Know the side effects of your/your patient's medicines:

Some medicines cause drowsiness, and still others cause sleeplessness. Some have to be taken with food and may produce adverse effects if not taken properly.

Keeping medicines out of the reach of children

Place them on a metal tray. Remove it from sight when children come to visit.

There are also changes that will need to be made to the home.

Items that the patient will use should be placed waist high or as close to that as possible. You may want to purchase grabbers so that patients don't have to reach or stoop. For the bathroom, tub bars and special commodes may be needed. A handheld sprayer for the shower is a wise investment as well.

Special Permit Parking

Most critically-ill patients will qualify for a handicapped parking sticker. This will prove beneficial when going to doctors' appointments, hospital trips, and pharmacy visits. To obtain a sticker (in some cities), get a statement from the attending physician which you can take to the Bureau of Motor Vehicles. For a small fee you will get a sticker to hang over the rear-view mirror. Be advised, however, that handicapped parking and wheelchair parking are two different things. The wheelchair spots are wider to allow for a wheelchair to enter and exit the vehicle.

Scriptural Reference:

> And, behold, a woman, which was diseased with an issue of blood twelve years, came behind him, and touched the hem of his garment. For she said within herself, If I may but touch his garment, I shall be whole.
>
> Matthew 9:20-21

CHAPTER 7

▼

HOLIDAYS AND
DEPRESSION

I can recall a sad event from the 1980s. A co-worker's mother died, and she decided to have the funeral on Thanksgiving Day. I had never heard of such a thing and didn't even realize that funeral homes were open on major holidays. I've often wondered if someone could have persuaded my co-worker to have the home-going services on another day. I would hate to mark holidays with that thought hanging heavily in the air.

It has been said that the holiday season brings bouts of extreme depression to a large number of people. For the chronically ill it presents a special challenge. Most people don't like a lot of noise and/or activity when they don't feel well. This is especially true of people who are heavily medicated, and are in all likelihood having moods swings.

Even if the patient is alert and not in pain, there's the financial side of the commercialized holidays. When a person is spending hundreds of dollars just to regulate their blood pressure and prevent seizures, there's not much left for shopping for gifts. This causes stress and hopelessness. The sick person's disabilities are magnified by all of the holiday hoopla. Joe was so hurt when his doctor told him not to get up on the ladder to decorate the outside of the house. He had already attempted the job before I told her. She insisted that he stop climbing ladders since his balance was poor. He was told to avoid anything that might cause a fall.

For the caregiver holidays are equally trying as the need to shop and prepare the house for guests is overshadowed by the constant care for the patient. The caregiver should, and must, take time to relax and unwind.

Things to Think About:
Establishing a Support Network

If there are no family members, perhaps there are friends and/or neighbors who will help out. Don't be too proud to accept help. There are centers which will care for an elderly or sick person for short periods during the day. Here in Indiana there are places called Board Care, Adult Foster Care, and Adult Family Care. Once called adult day-care facilities, the stigma often attached to them has been erased. To provide care for adults, it is not necessary to get a license if you have fewer than five non-related members in your home. Since there are more than 30,000 people on waiting lists for home health care in Indiana, area churches are putting together programs which offer assistance. And nursing homes are even using parts of their facilities to accommodate adults who need care during various periods of the day.

Even minimum assistance would provide an opportune time for the caregiver to spend time relaxing, working out at a gym, going to a movie, or maybe even a spa! Get an appointment for a body wrap, a massage, manicure, and pedicure. Spa's are great for men as well as women! It is important that the caregiver pamper himself/herself somewhat so as not to become too stressed out. Proper diet and exercise is just as important for the caregiver as for the patient.

Read comforting passages and stories

The "Good Shepherd" John 10:1-16

The term shepherd is mentioned in the following 17 books of the Bible: Genesis, Numbers, I Samuel, I Kings, II Chronicles, Psalms, Ecclesiastes, Isaiah, Jeremiah, Ezekiel, Amos, Zechariah, Matthew, Mark, John, Hebrews, and I Peter. The predominate theme throughout is that the congregation is in need of a shepherd. There is a scattering of the flock. Numbers 27:17 compares a congregation of the Lord with sheep without a shepherd.

Which may go out before them, and which may go in before them, and which may lead them out, and which may bring them in; that the congregation of the Lord be not as sheep which have no shepherd. (Numbers 27:17).

The terms *Chief Shepherd* and *Great Shepherd* are used in various biblical scriptures, but the term *Good Shepherd* is used only once, and that is by Christ in John 10:11. Christ says that thieves and robbers try to enter the sheepfold by climbing the wall. In this passage Christ is referring to Jewish leaders. Christ goes on to say that the true leader enters by the door and is the only shepherd. The sheep follow the true shepherd; he calls them by name; they hear his voice, and they respond knowing his voice.

> The Lord is my shepherd, I shall not want. He maketh me to lie down in green pastures. He leadeth me beside the still waters. He restoreth my soul. He leadeth me in the paths of righteousness for His name sake. Yea, thou I walk through the valley of the shadow of death, I will fear no evil. For thou art with me. Thy rod and thy staff they comfort me. Thou prepareth a table before me in the presence of mine enemies. My cup runneth over. Surely goodness and mercy shall follow me, all the days of my life. And I shall dwell in the house of the Lord, forever.

Psalm 23

Scriptural Reference:

> These things I have spoken unto you, that in me ye might have peace. In the world ye shall have tribulation: but be of good cheer; I have overcome the world.

John 16:33

CHAPTER 8

▼

TAKING CARE OF BUSINESS/WHOM TO NOTIFY

For some caregivers the chore of managing the patient will be coupled with handling the finances of the loved one. This can be a touchy area, as some people, no matter how ill, don't relish the thought of someone else having control of all of their financial business.

If someone asks you to take a check to the bank or make a car payment, the average person wouldn't think twice. But when the stroke victim is not able to answer calls from creditors, other problems will be encountered. Due to the privacy laws, creditors are not allowed to reveal payment history and/or other details about accounts to anyone other than the party to whom credit was extended.

At that juncture it is advisable to consult an attorney and arrange for Power of Attorney. That will allow the caregiver to make medical and financial decisions.

Things to Think About

During the moments when the patient is depressed and/or despondent, try to show him/her that you sincerely care about them. This probably can't be stressed enough.

A Flower for the Living

I would rather have a little rose
From the garden of a friend,
Than flowers strewn around my casket
When my days on earth must end.
I would rather have a living smile
From one I know is true
Than tears shed 'round my casket
When this world I bid adieu.
Bring me all the flowers today
Whether pink or white or red;
I would rather have one blossom now
Than a truckload when I'm dead.

Author Unknown

Scriptural Reference:
The following scripture is good for the patient and the caregiver.

> But he that knew not, and did commit things worthy of stripes, shall be beaten with few stripes. For unto whomsoever much is given, of him shall be much required: and to whom men have committed much, of him they will ask the more.

Luke 16:22

CHAPTER 9

▼

DUE TIME/FAITH

Divine Appointment: A Caregiver's Guide wouldn't be complete without a chapter on death and grieving. Even though all sickness is not unto death, surely we all know that dying is a necessary part of life. Things will eventually come to an end in due time, even Eschatology—the doctrine of Last Things! When the end is near, people start speculating about time. How many days? How many weeks? How many months? How many years? The answer to all of those questions lies with the ONE who gave life in the first place. We are a people obsessed with time, albeit *chronos*, or sequential time. We want God to honor this system, but he has his own. He operates on *kairos*, a special time that is in God's *Fullness of Time*.

The important thing for all of us to do is to prepare for death. We shouldn't leave this very necessary part of our life for someone else to do! Since it is a painful topic of discussion for people who are ill, we should make a conscious decision to handle our business while we have use of all of our faculties. One wise thing would be to make pre-arrangements, which means planning things out. You can even have unfunded pre-arrangements, where the funeral home of your choice will keep a record of all of your requests. Keep in mind that you can't pre-arrange burial plots at the cemetery without payment. It is wise to decide on a funeral home, and what you want done to your body before disposition takes place. The funeral home is happy to keep this on record! Then when we trade time for eternity, all will be in order. Of course your family will still have to pay for the charges incurred by the funeral home and the cemetery.

When a Loved One Dies at Home

If there are machines (ventilators, monitors, and others) attached to the deceased, ask a doctor or nurse to remove them before the mortician comes to pick up the body. Lubricate the face lightly with Vaseline, paying special attention to the areas above the eyes and the lips. These are the moisture areas that will dry out quickly. Since you don't know the exact time that the mortician will arrive, the moisture you can retain in the body will help a lot. If the deceased had been wearing dentures in the previous week or two, put them back in. If he/she had not worn them for a month, don't attempt to put them in; an embalmer will use a *mouth former*. But take the deceased's dentures to the funeral home and let them decide on how they want to handle the situation.

Try to straighten out the body, close the mouth, open the hands and place the deceased in a supine position. They will sometimes put themselves in awkward positions when death is imminent. They may put their hands on their face, ball their fists, or even get in a fetal position. Once rigor mortis sets in, it is hard to straighten out the body.

If there is hair on the face, let the mortician know if you want it to stay. Some men and women look natural with facial hair, so make sure that the person picking up the body has your wishes written down so they can relay that information to the embalmer or mortician.

If the deceased had been under a doctor's care or hospice, call the last physician, and he will sign the death certificate later on. The physician will tell you to call your funeral home to pick up the body. If the deceased was not under care, call 911, and the coroner will make the pronouncement of death. If the coroner suspects foul play, he will send the body to the morgue. In a more routine situation he will sign the release of the body and allow you to call your funeral home. An EMT (an emergency medical technician who responds to the 911 call) cannot make the death pronouncement!

When you call a funeral home, a director will call the family back to formalize, get permission to embalm, and set up an appointment. Something to remember when planning the date of the services:

- Don't give anyone dates until the services have been finalized

- When people are notified of the date of services, they plan to be off work, and some even have to travel from out of town. This presents a hardship when the date they were given proves to be incorrect.

- You might have a date in mind, but the funeral home might not be able to accommodate you.

In the Hospital

If you know that a patient is terminally ill, you should call a funeral home to find out what you need to do when death occurs. You need not make a decision until after the death of the patient. When death occurs, tell the hospital staff that you have made a choice in a funeral home, and they will notify them to come and pick up the body. Some hospitals have the family sign a release form when the patient dies. Other hospitals might require the family to go to the funeral home of their choice to sign the release form. Then the funeral home will pick up the body. Although you don't want to take a lot of time deciding where the body will go, you don't have to make a decision right at the point of death!

In funded or unfunded pre-arrangements, designate a family member and let them know where papers are. Patients on heavy medication and elderly patients should take someone with them when making arrangements. Bear in mind that there are some unscrupulous funeral homes. When planning to do business with a funeral home, make sure you contact the Better Business Bureau and/or the National Funeral Directors Association. Some people have reported horror stories wherein they paid for pre-arranged services for loved ones, but the prices were hiked when time for the funeral arrived.

Coroner's Case

If there are questionable circumstances surrounding the death, the coroner will become involved. In that case the family will have to go to the funeral home to sign the release form in order for that funeral home to pick up the body.

Trustee Case

In the event that there is no money for burial, the matter becomes a *Trustee case*. When you call the funeral home, inform them that this will be a Trustee case. Some funeral homes will not pick up the body until they know that it is a confirmed Trustee case. The Trustee's Office in some states will only offer cremation or immediate burial with a cloth-covered casket. In Indiana they will pay $600.00 toward the funeral home charges and $400.00 for the burial. Since you are declaring that you have no money, you are not free to upgrade this service. That is, the Trustee is not supposed to accept money from the family!

Medicaid Case

In Indiana Medicaid will apply $400 toward the funeral charges, and the family is allowed to contribute up to $750. The total allowable cost for a funeral in Indiana, paid for under the Medicaid guidelines, is $1,150. Check with the funeral home of your choice to see if they accept Trustee and/or Medicaid cases. If you have a body sent to a funeral home that does not accept Trustee or Medicaid cases, you will have the added inconvenience of having the body moved to another funeral home. Ask the funeral home what services they provide for Trustee and Medicaid cases.

Planning a Home-going Ceremony

This task can be painless if you plan in advance. People should do this when they are well. Then it's not so depressing. Prepare a list of family, friends, and advisors. Jot their addresses and phone numbers down in a safe place. If you have a preference for a church, note that, along with the order of service you'd like. Below is a list of things to do for those left behind, (It would behoove us all to plan this as much as possible, before that time comes.)

People to Notify

> The Cemetery
>
> Unions
>
> Social Organizations
>
> Military Service
>
> Insurance Agents
>
> Minister and Church
>
> Pianist/Choir Director or Soloist
>
> Newspapers

At the time of death there are certain arrangements which have to be made. A survivor will be required to supply the deceased's vital statistics to the State, to obtain a death certificate. The information for the obituary will be needed if not already done. Make sure to list all schools the deceased attended. There may also be the need for a list of pallbearers, flower girls, and a line-up of friends and family for the procession. The left behind will have to: answer calls from those extending sympathy, go to the funeral home to make the arrangements, provide information and directions to the services, receive out-of-town guests, and keep up with letters, cards, and other condolences. There is also the case of deciding where the dinner will be held (if applicable).

The wise person will even purchase their burial plot well in advance. Of course there will be additional charges, such as the opening and closing of the burial plot, the cost of the casket, the interment service, the funeral director's fee, the church (in most instances), and the police escorts (if available).

Oftentimes the family doesn't purchase the marker during the arrangements but instead will wait until later. The markers may be flat or raised, and you may also choose to have a monument, which is normally in reference to the family. It's sentimental and contains language of a personal nature. Markers and monuments have to be ordered, and it usually takes several weeks for delivery.

Example of an Obituary

"For I am now ready to be offered, and the time of my departure is at hand. I have fought a good fight, I have finished my course, I have kept the faith." (II Timothy 4:6-7)

Delores Jean Lewis, daughter of Chester and Daisy Lewis, was born on August 12, 1949, in Indianapolis, Indiana. At an early age she professed a hope in Christ and was baptized. She was united in marriage to Roy Thomas Offett. Delores attended schools in Indianapolis and graduated from Indiana Business College in 1974. She was a member of the U.S. Army Reserves (assigned to 425th PSC, Indianapolis) and was honorably discharged in 1978. She later married Walter William Thornton, Jr., and to this union one child was born.

Delores attended Simmons Baptist Bible College, Indianapolis Extension, majoring in Christian Education. A retired postal worker (1973-2003), she served in the following capacities: clerk, job instructor, union steward, and coordinator for various programs. An author with a vision, she founded Marguerite Press, Marguerite Press Promo, and was a literacy volunteer for Indy Reads. She was also the host of the syndicated Internet radio show *Around2it*.

Delores was preceded in death by her Father, Chester Lewis; sister, Annette Louise Lewis; brothers, Dennis Kelvin, and William Maurice Lewis. She leaves to mourn her passing: Mother, Daisy B. Lewis. Daughters: Dana, Monica, Rhonda (Lamont), and Alta. Grandchildren: Eboni, William, Cameron, Brittany, Jasmine and Myles. Sisters: Constance Clark, Shirley Bailey, Gloria Vaughn, Deborah Kendall, Lana Talib, Linda Everett. Brothers: Chester, Rudolph Alfred, and James Lewis. Special Friends, Joe Nathan Clark, Lena Williams, Gloria Oliver, and a host of other relatives and friends.

WHEN THE MOURNING COMES
by Delores Thornton

Please don't weep or mourn for me
As if I died today,
For I laid down my yoke
and simply passed away;
I wish that I could comfort you
And bring smiles through all your tears,
But rest assured that I'm okay;
There are no problems here.
When you think of me, as you will do,
Put a smile upon your face,
And remember I love you, and I am not dead,
Just in a better place.

Humbly submitted   The Family

Example of a Home-going Ceremony

Order of Service:

Processional	Soft Music
Prayer	
Scripture	
Solo	*Trouble of the World*
Acknowledgments	Church Clerk
Obituary	Read Silently
Solo	*His Eye is on the Sparrow*
Remarks	
Words of Comfort	Rev. Joy L. Thornton
Review	(Solo) *The Last Mile of the Way*
Benediction	

Recessional

Committal & Interment   Crown Hill Cemetery

*   *   *   *

Appreciation

The family wishes to acknowledge with deep appreciation the many comforting messages, prayers, and many other expressions of kindness. You will receive a more formal thank you at a later time. May God richly bless you.

Pallbearers

Dana Elmore	Monica Elmore
Rhonda Perry	Lamont Perry
Alta Thornton	Eboni Elmore

Honorary Pallbearers

William Elmore	Brittany Elmore
Cameron Elmore	James Lewis

A Newspaper Obituary

The preceding obituary is an example of the type found on the program, but there is another type for the press. Newspapers provide a free death notice which includes: name, age, and residence of the deceased. For an additional fee, a list of survivors and a photograph of the deceased may be added.

When the Deceased is a Veteran

As previously stated, it is advisable to inform your funeral home if the deceased was a veteran. There are certain benefits for active and honorably discharged members of the armed forces. The funeral home will obtain a U.S. flag and make arrangements for Military Funeral Honors to send a bereavement team which will fold the flag. Additionally, the team will either do a live presentation of *Taps* or will play a recording.

What to do After the Home-going Ceremony

Remember that faith in God will sustain you during all of the seasons of your life.

- Meditate and Pray.

  And Naomi said to her daughter-in-law, Blessed be he of the Lord, who hath not left off his kindness to the living and to the dead. And Naomi said unto her, the man is near of kin unto us, one of our next kinsmen. Ruth 2:20

- Pay any left-over bills.

- Send cards of thanks to all of the well-wishers.

- *Distribute flowers and plants to nursing homes (or to friends and family).*

- Apply for survivor's benefits (if deceased was a spouse). For more information on Social Security Benefits, contact the administration at: 1-800-234-5772. For Veteran's Benefits call, 1-202-872-1151.

For Society Security Benefits remember to have:

Social Security Number

Death Certificate

Birth Certificate

Marriage Certificate

Paid Invoices from the Funeral Home

Birth Certificates for children under 18

For Veteran's Benefits remember to have:

A copy of the honorably discharged veterans' Death Certificate

Paid invoices from the Funeral Home

Birth Certificates of all children under 18

Copy of the Marriage License

Copy of the Discharge papers (DD214)

Things to Think About

There are numerous cemeteries which have become full service, or *combo's*. They have a chapel in which the funeral is held. It is of course conveniently located near the gravesite which eliminates the need for a procession, and in some cases it simplifies the organizing of services. Combo's are separate entities which share the same grounds. Since families have to visit the funeral home and the cemetery while ordering services, this idea of combining the two is a beneficial for some families. Some, however, still desire the more traditional *church home-going ceremony*. For this reason families may, for an additional fee, request a church service from their combo provider.

The Interview with God

I dreamed I had an interview with God.

"So you would like to interview me?" God asked.

"If you have the time," I said.

God smiled. "My time is eternity."
"What questions do you have in mind for me?"

"What surprises you most about humankind?"

God answered…
"That they get bored with childhood,
they rush to grow up, and then
long to be children again.

That they lose their health to make money…
and then lose their money to restore their health.

That by thinking anxiously about the future,
they forget the present,
such that they live in neither
the present nor the future.

That they live as if they will never die,
and die as though they had never lived."

God's hand took mine,
and we were silent for a while.

And then I asked…
"As a parent, what are some of life's lessons
you want your children to learn?"

"To learn they cannot make anyone
love them. All they can do
is let themselves be loved.

"To learn that it is not good
to compare themselves to others.

"To learn to forgive
by practicing forgiveness.

"To learn that it only takes a few seconds
to open profound wounds in those they love,
and it can take many years to heal them.

"To learn that a rich person
is not one who has the most,
but is one who needs the least.

"To learn that there are people
who love them dearly,
but simply have not yet learned
how to express or show their feelings.

"To learn that two people can
look at the same thing
and see it differently.

"To learn that it is not enough that they
forgive one another, but they must also forgive themselves."

"Thank you for your time," I said humbly.

"Is there anything else
you would like your children to know?"

God smiled and said,
"Just know that I am here…always."

Author unknown

Scriptural Reference:

> But of that day and that hour knoweth no man, no, not the angels which are
> in heaven, neither the Son, but the Father.
> Take ye heed, watch and pray; for ye know not when the time is.

Mark 13:32-33

CHAPTER 10

▼

GUS/STEPPING OUT OF THE BOWL

It is such a testimony when people recover from grave illnesses. Joe no longer has to go to the speech therapist. And he can swallow clear liquids without the aid of thickeners. He still has a slight limp and must walk with a cane, but, thank God, he is still in the land of the living. Although he still needs special care, it feels good to have time to myself—time to dream dreams, and work to make them come true. It's almost like stepping out of the bowl.

*   *   *   *

A Goldfish Named Gus

It is a pleasure to remember a simpler taste of life, like back when the local five and dime stores, G. C. Murphy's and F.W. Woolworth's, gave youngsters baby chicks during the Easter holidays. Most of the time the tiny birds wouldn't live more than a few weeks, but the furry fuzzy birds brought tons of joy to area children. In the mid-1950s, the Board of Health outlawed the sale of chicks in the city limits. During that same period the Indiana State Fair was offering goldfish as a prize for the ring toss. Usually the little helpless creatures died before they reached their respective homes. The tiny baggies were either dropped, and the water poured out, or they just died.

In 1988 my grandchildren won two goldfish at the fair. Their eyes were as wide as saucers when they showed me their winnings. They even named them. Of the two, one name escapes me, but one fish had the name Gus. One fish was dead the next morning, but Gus lived for many years.

Gus lived although the kids often overfed him, ignoring my instruction to place a few breadcrumbs in the bowl so he wouldn't overeat. Gus lived although we sometimes took vacations and forgot to feed him at all. Gus even survived a move in sub-zero temperatures when we left our old home and lived in an apartment while awaiting construction of our new house.

Gus gave our family plenty of hours of excitement as we sat around the bowl and watched him swish and splash throughout the day. He was really a family pet. What was so amazing about Gus was that he could survive outside of his fishbowl. I often wondered if he even knew he was a goldfish! Once I came home and found him outside of his bowl, just lying on the top of the stove. Another time he was in the middle of the kitchen floor. Gus had more lives than a cat it seemed, and it always surprised us to see him still alive out of his natural environment. It got to the point that when we entered the house we'd look down to avoid stepping on him, and I'd carefully inspect the stovetop before turning it on. We always tread lightly until we came to Gus' bowl and found him inside.

Gus died in 1995, and though we didn't know anything about the longevity of goldfish, my family and I were sure that Gus had set a record. At least a record for State Fair goldfish!

No one knows how long they have. Some lives are sadly short, like the no-name fish. Some live on against all odds and in the face of great adversity like Gus. The important thing is to not give in too easily, for God helps us think outside the bowl!

Scripture Reference:

> But they that wait upon the Lord shall renew their strength; they shall mount up with wings as eagles; they shall run, and not be weary; and they shall walk, and not faint.

> Isaiah 40:31

CHAPTER 11

▼

JOSEPH'S STORY/WHEN THE PATIENT IS A CHILD

In this chapter we are going to hear from nine-year-old Joseph Kierre Carr. Since Joseph has never spoken before, you have to listen very closely to grasp the meaning of his love!

My name is Joseph Kierre Carr, and I'm nine year's old. I was born with a condition called Schizencephaly, a form of Cerebral Palsy. My brain has clefts which didn't form properly. My condition caused a developmental delay and severe mental retardation. There is no known cause and no cure.

In a typical day my Mom, Kenya Carr, bathes me, checks the site of my feeding tube for leakage, then gives me my medicine. Next Mom dresses me. I've had the feeding tube for seven years, and I must be administered food through it twice a day, once in the morning and again at night. Next my Mom gets my equipment ready. I have a *standard* in which I stand. This strengthens and supports my legs. After breakfast Mom gets the splints and braces ready, then places me in my wheelchair.

I go to daycare from 6:30-9:00 a.m. Then a bus picks me up and takes me to school. I attend Indianapolis Public School #48 where I get therapy. I'm in a Special Education Class, and I enjoy working with clay with the aid of my teachers. Once a year Mom comes to my school to help set goals for my therapy, and my report card reflects how I've met those goals.

At the end of the school day Mom takes me home and fixes dinner for my brother Julian and herself. Julian is only four years old, but he's very active. Julian and I love each other very much! Mom checks my briefs (Depends), then gives me range of motion exercises.

At night Mom bathes me, checks my feeding tube, and prepares me for bed. I have to wear a *bi-pap* which gives oxygen because I have the tendency to pull my tongue back, and that blocks my airways. I also have a nighttime feeding tube. Although I normally sleep through the night, I sometimes have laughing spells. Laughing and crying are the only forms of communication I have.

I worry about my Mom sometimes, for as a single parent she has had an unusually hard time. I'm almost four feet tall, and I weigh sixty-eight pounds, so I know that it's physically hard for her to lift me as much as she does. There have been times when it was difficult to maneuver my wheelchair, but thank goodness the city has really improved in making places more accessible, and it is now easier to navigate city streets. At a birthday party recently a few men at the mall had to carry me and my wheelchair up a flight of stairs since there was no elevator. And there have been times when my family couldn't attend events, for Mom didn't have the money to pay for a box seat to accommodate my wheelchair.

There is also the case of emotional strain on Mom, and I sometimes think she's in a state of denial. She probably feels like she's been on a bus ride and gotten off at the wrong stop, and everything is unfamiliar. I'm glad she has a support network, although she's a strong independent woman and doesn't seek help often. She only leaves me with my Aunt Connie or my Grandma Debra, and then only for brief periods of time.

I'm optimistic to a certain extent! I've had so many surgeries until I can't say how many, but my last one was two years ago. When I was hospitalized, my Mom stayed with me the entire time, and she was satisfied with my quality of care. I'm also on an oral medicine, and in January 2004, my doctor said my muscles were more loose, and I may not have to get additional medicines. I don't get sick as much as I once did, so Mom doesn't have to leave work as often as she once did.

Mom used to worry about a life insurance policy for me, thinking she'd have to borrow against her own policy when the time came. No insurance company would issue her a policy since I'm considered a high risk. Mom recently found out that she'll be eligible for assistance when the need arises, and that put her mind to rest.

I'm considered a special needs child, and I don't have a problem with that. I'm just so happy that I was sent to a special person! Mom, I love you.

Things to think about:
Kenya's Bio

Joseph's story was narrated by Kenya Carr, a Coding Support Clerk at an Indianapolis hospital. She's been employed there for nine years and currently works in a section with nine other workers. Though Kenya rarely goes out, when she does she likes to take in a good movie or make a quick stop at a nightclub. An avid reader she enjoys romance, but she also curls up with mysteries and other nonfiction works.

As a single mom Kenya has to budget her time wisely, yet she still realizes it is important to have some "me time."

When the Patient is a Sibling

Georgena Anderson is an Indianapolis, Indiana, resident who has five siblings, one of whom is a forty-one year old sister, Rachel Johnson, who is mildly handicapped. At age three Rachel developed a form of meningitis, and it left her with symptoms of slow learning disability, poor reflexes, epilepsy, and scoliosis. She also has a speech impediment.

Rachel went to school to age twenty and was cared for by her parents until the 1980s when her mother died. A former resident of the state of Michigan, Rachel was rescued by Georgena who brought her to Indiana to live. She stayed with her sisters for a short time while awaiting an opening to move into a group home.

Georgena expressed frustration in battling state agencies over Rachel's rights. Georgena has had Power of Attorney for her sister in the past and is now her Health Care Representative. She went to the hospital when Rachel had problems with her neurological system or suffered numerous seizures. Rachel has been semi-independent for the past five years, and just recently (winter 2004) she moved into her own apartment. Other family members traveled from Michigan to help move her.

"It was a hassle at first," said Georgena. "The state had so many cutbacks that she had to find cheaper housing and living arrangements. A co-signer was also needed to secure her apartment, and unfortunately the agency which provides her services and receives her monies was not willing to assist."

Rachel receives twelve hours of care daily from a private agency which is licensed and regulated by the State of Indiana. She can cook and clean, but the care provider still offers valuable assistance with her day-to-day living skills. The care provider also takes Rachel shopping, helps her with laundry, and even joins her in arts and crafts projects. Rachel works twelve hours per week at her filing job and enjoys her freedom.

"She'll get a medic-alert next week," Georgena said. "She also does water aerobics, and I bought her an exercise bike. She needs a scooter because she falls about one hundred times a year due to her poor reflexes. The scooter costs $2,500, so for right now I just rent one when we go on our yearly vacations."

She looks to her family for some of the financial support, but it's not always easy. Families often disagree on the best course of action to take, especially when it is expensive or labor intensive. Georgena is grateful for the family members who have been consistent supporters of her efforts.

Georgena is Rachel's advocate. She speaks with the agency and state officials on her behalf throughout the year. She's even taped some sessions with officials so she could play them over and over as she explains to Rachel what was going on. Fortunately Rachel has Blue Cross insurance from her father's former employer, as well as Medicaid, so her quality of health care is sufficient.

Georgena says, "Parents hang in there with their children who have disabilities, but, if they can, it's important for them to make preparations for a disabled child's needs after they leave this earth. And it's not just a question of who can financially support a disabled son, daughter, or sibling, but rather who can best provide the love and commitment to do it."

Scriptural Reference:

> And now abideth faith, hope, charity, these three; but the greatest of these is charity.

I Corinthians 13:13

CHAPTER 12

▼

WHEN THE PATIENT IS A PARENT

I met MarshaRose Joyner a short time ago, but it's as if we've known each other longer. While working on this book I asked others to share their experiences. MarshaRose responded with this heart-wrenching story of Dr. Elizabeth Murphy Oliver Abney.

Taking Care of Mom

So here I am, in the autumn of my life, having said goodbye to my mother. It is difficult to convey the immeasurable memories of her—an unmovable force, the rock solid foundation of my life.

Mama, my mother, Dr. Elizabeth Murphy Oliver Abney. The most indomitable spirit I have ever known. With skin like warm brown velvet and charm that belied her legendary unconquerable toughness. Her spirit so commanding. Her words so powerfully persuasive. She was a tiny woman, yet she loomed over everything and everyone she touched.

Christmas Eve, 1998, and no telephone call from Mama. How strange! She never missed a day like this. Mama loved holidays—the cards, the colors, and the music that connotes the season. Christmas day I called her, and still no response. How could she miss Christmas? I had mailed a package to her and knew she would call when it was received. I called and called for three days and no response. Where could she be?

Finally I called my cousin Jake Oliver (publisher of the Afro-American Newspapers). "Where is Mama?…What do you mean she is not with you?" As I raised my voice several octaves, "Christmas! And you do not know where she is? This is December 27, and you do not know where @$* she is!?" The six thousand miles seemed worlds away. I called the police in Baltimore at the same time Jake did. They arrived to find her lying on the floor where she had been since December 24.

"Honey Bun, I could hear the phone, but could not reach it. That is how I knew I was alive," Mama whispered to me as Jake held the phone. Soon the ambulance came to take her to the hospital.

In the length of that phone call life changed. My daughter Marilyn and I left Hawaii for Baltimore to get Mama.

That January had to have been the coldest winter on record. Or so it seemed to me, not having lived in cold weather for thirty years. The Catholic Mercy Hospital was at the bottom of the hill from Mama's Charles Plaza condo, across the street from a magnificent cathedral, the first Catholic Diocese in America, established 1789. When I was a child, this area of Baltimore was so beautiful. The seemingly anachronistic tradition of Flower Mart, held the first Tuesday in May, had charmed Baltimoreans since 1915. Not even two world wars prevented the whole affair from going off without a hitch on the streets and squares surrounding the Washington Monument, the first such monument, Baltimoreans were proud to note, in Mt. Vernon Place. Mama loved living in this area. It was almost safe. As a child walking in the cold and snow, Mama would tell me about that old drafty house in Baltimore, the home of Edgar Allen Poe's Annabelle Lee.

January 6, 1999, in the most beautiful and frightening ice storm I have ever witnessed, Marilyn and I walked down to the hospital laughing and giggling, holding hands, picking our way through the ice and snow, step by step we descended through the terraced Mt. Vernon Park that lies between Charles Place and the hospital. From out of nowhere two men, who were a picture perfect replica of "street people," dressed in torn and tattered clothing, one tall, slender, scruffy white man and a shorter, rounder Black man came up to us and smiled broadly. In all of two seconds we made the decision to return the smile.

"Ladies, may we help you through the ice and snow?"

Marilyn and I looked at each other and in one voice replied, "Why not?'

So our white, tall, slender, scruffy gentleman bowed low in his best Sir Walter Raleigh gesture, put out his three quarter gloved hand while the shorter, rounder

Black man came around on the other side, and we proceeded through the misery without missing a step. In two minutes we were at the hospital. They opened the door and ushered us in. Then they vanished as quickly as they had appeared. Not giving another thought to them, we brushed off the snow and rode in silence on the full elevator to see Mama.

The next day was just as cold and just as miserable. We left One Charles Place to see Mama, and our Sir Walter Raleighs were sitting on a bench. We waved and swiftly stayed the course of our journey. We were in the badlands of Baltimore for three weeks, and every time we ventured forth, they were there…our Sir Walter Raleighs…just there…they would wave and smile…they were there.

"Your mother can no longer live alone. She has emphysema, and her legs are not sturdy. She requires constant care," the doctor said. "What nursing home do you want to send her to?"

"My home is where she is going," I answered.

"Hawaii? All the way to Hawaii?" the doctor asked.

"Yes, I have her ticket, and we are leaving soon."

Marilyn and I began the arduous task of cataloguing and distributing her belongings to the Schomburg Museum, family and friends. My entire life unfolded before me. Mama had kept everything—it was a joyous adventure with my daughter into the past. We were like little kids playing grownup. I had always wanted to explore Mama's closets and drawers. She had such marvelous things. Pictures of great people, baby pictures, family pictures that stretched back to the 1800's, Civil Rights Movement pictures, pictures of her 40 years at the Afro-American newspapers. You name it, she had a picture of it: 5,000 pictures (by actual count), Christmas cards from famous people, antique jewelry, telephone bills from her mother in Brazil, Indiana (where we were born), luxurious fur coats, crystal chandeliers, out of print magazines, and 800 books.

Everyday Marilyn and I would walk down the hill in the snow and ice to the hospital. Everyday the staff would ask if we were going to take her home.

"Not yet," we replied.

I knew if Mama suspected what we were up to, it would never happen. After three weeks of packing, shipping, and closing her home, we picked her up at the hospital and went straight to the airport. There waiting for us was a group of her friends and relatives to say goodbye.

Traveling with oxygen tanks, a wheelchair, carry-on bags, etc., for ten hours is an adventure in itself. However, we had made arrangements with the airline in advance, so they were ready for us. The pilot announced that we would be flying with oxygen on board, so if anyone had an issue, to please let him know. Instead of issues there was love—the other passengers pitched in and made it comfortable.

I delighted in the turn of events. For the 60 years I had been on this planet, Mama had been totally in control. Now the roles were reversed. I could take care of and love her as I wished to do for so long.

My husband Kenneth gave up his privacy and transformed his office into a room for Mama. He installed a hospital bed with lots of pillows and pretty linens, familiar pictures on the wall, and an oversized television. The drone of the oxygen generator just outside the bedroom door was to become the background of our lives.

Life was new. Each day was a learning experience. I believe I expected her to get better in the Hawaiian sunshine and fresh air. But it did not happen. Friends with experience, and those without, came to help with Mama's care. The First Church of Christian Science sent stacks of videotapes because that had been her practice for many, many years.

The days melted into nights, and our home became a busy place of abode with the constant comings and goings. She became "Mama" to everyone. And everyone supplied love, comfort, and support.

Of all of the years I had known my mother, this was the first time she had surrendered. Well, almost! There was the night when she had almost stopped breathing, and we called the paramedics. For hours Mama put up a fight—she was not going to the hospital. "They kill people in there!" Mama announced in her commanding voice. "I'm not going. I know my rights, and I'm not going anywhere with you."

This went on for the better part of two hours. The paramedics called the police to witness that she was refusing to allow them to take her to the hospital. If she were to die, they did not want to be sued.

"I've never seen anything this like in my life," one of the medics said.

Well, you cannot blame her. In 1914 when Mama was born, the world was filled with a hatred called Jim Crow. In Brazil, Indiana, her father, Dr. Jacob B. Oliver, was the only doctor in that little town, and that made life secure. However, everyone knew of the existence of the KKK. Going away to college at Fisk University in the 1930's, Mama said there was a lynching just outside of Nashville every weekend. One could feel the hatred in the air.

So no, she was not going with these strange men to a hospital with people whose faces were foreign to her.

Kenneth and Mama's relationship deepened and bloomed. He gave his all to her care. They had long conversations and shared many tender moments. Then he would come out of her room and cry. He cooked for her and shopped for her. There was nothing Mama wanted for that he did not make every attempt to secure. "I began to feel like she was my mother," Ken said. "I could not have done any more if she was."

Watching this strong woman fade away while laboring for every breath, listening to the drone of the oxygen, smelling the antiseptic, enduring daily laundry and sleepless nights, and knowing there was nothing I could do to stop the process was so difficult. Taking charge, acting like I was in control, and never letting Mama see me cry—it was the love of everyone around us that got me through it all.

August 11 1999, midnight

I had made a big deal, as only I can make a big deal, of Mama being with me when I took my first breath, so I needed to be with her when she took her last. Today we were alone. For some reason no hospice people, no Kenneth, no volunteers, just the two of us. So I crawled into bed with Mama and drifted into a deep and comforting sleep. At 4:00 p.m. the telephone rang. I made no attempt to answer it. Looking up at the clock and making a mental note of the time, I took Mama's hand in mine and just lay there. At 4:07 Mama breathed deep, and it was her last.

The hospice nurse gave instructions *not* to call the police or the coroner's office. They just complicate matters, and instead of a precious time, a memorial point in time, death becomes a bureaucratic nightmare.

The hospice people were on their way. Judith anointed Mama with lovely oils, and I dressed her in a pretty pink gown. Her face softened as all of the pain and hurts were gone. One of the hospice nurses brought fresh flowers for her room. Juliet arrived with a lei the same color as the dainty flowers in the linens. The room was a picture of loveliness.

On the phone I asked the funeral home how long could I keep Mama before they had to come get her to prepare for cremation. "Midnight it will be."

Immediately we held an exquisite bedside service with all of the family, friends, and hospice people in attendance. The hospice minister, who had become such an integral part of our daily routine, prayed; the contralto voice of the hospice practical nurse left not a dry eye in the place as people shared their special feelings about being there in that marvelous moment. Death was welcomed; the suffering was over, and passing was beautiful.

I sat alone, recording all of the details of the day in my memory banks, when suddenly Mama appeared as regal and beautiful as I can recall, glowing from within and clothed in a beautiful pink gown. Peering through the tears, I said goodbye, and she was gone.

At midnight two men arrived dressed in white, one tall, slender white man and one shorter, rounder Black man—they gently removed Mama and smiled at me and bowed low—these were the same faces of our Sir Walter Raleigh's! Years later Marilyn and I agreed we had met our guardian angels.

Elizabeth Murphy Oliver, Ph.D., my mother, went to work at the Afro-American Newspapers October 1941. Hers was the sixth generation of an African American family which dates back to 1740. She was born to Dr. Jacob B. Oliver of Brazil, Indiana, (who was born a slave) and Rose Murphy Oliver of Baltimore, Maryland, daughter of Afro-American Newspapers founder, John H. Murphy, Sr.

In the 40 years she was in the newspapers industry, having been born into it, Dr. Oliver collected more than 5,000 pictures and documents depicting Black Heritage. She was awarded the "Black Marylanders of Distinction Award" along with 91 other awards for her continued work on behalf of the African-American community. She was named a "Living Legend" by The Schomburg Museum, New York City Library.

Elizabeth Murphy Oliver is survived by her only daughter, MarshaRose Joyner, President of the Dr. Martin Luther King, Jr. Holiday Coalition, and her son-in-law, Kenneth R. Joyner, owner of the Hair Fair Beauty Salon in the Edgewater Hotel, Waikiki, Hawaii; a granddaughter, Marilyn Carter, Wai'anae, Hawaii; grandsons Elmer Wesley III, Honolulu; Christopher Marshall German, San Francisco; Gregory Stuart German, Berkeley, California; and four great-grand children, Shaina Carter, Ashley Amber Amps, Andrew and Aaron Amps, of Honolulu.

We had the privilege of keep and caring for Mama in her last days on earth. For a motto to live by, I must quote my husband. "Everyday you wake up is a good day." Gawd dun smile pun we!

"Gawd dun smile pun we!" comes from the Gullah Islands of South Carolina, and it means God has blessed us.

*   *   *   *

Blessed to Have Her with Us

The following are words from Janet Lewis. I interviewed Janet, and this is her story:

*   *   *   *

My mother, Agnes Rowlette, is an Indianapolis native and current resident. In 1991 she suffered a light stroke. Mom and I had lived together for years, and it really took me by surprise; prior to that she'd only been relatively healthy. She had been diagnosed with diabetes, but it was under control. Though I was upset, somehow I managed to drive Mom to the hospital. The stroke affected her speech and her left hand. Her face also became twisted, and she developed a limp.

Mom was hospitalized for about a week, but fortunately for her there was an experimental drug being introduced for stroke victims. She had to sign numerous papers, and my siblings and I had to sign them as well. Under the guidance of the doctors she participated in a study. Her recovery was no less than miraculous. Her face returned to its natural shape, her walk improved, and her speech improved.

The doctors were so pleased with her progress that they filmed a television commercial featuring her. The commercial aired on local channels in the Indianapolis area.

It has been almost 15 years since the stroke, and Mom continues to improve. She is not on any medicines for high blood pressure, but she is on medication and a special diet for her diabetes. My six siblings and I realize that we are blessed to still have Mom with us, and since she's retired, she is content to enjoy her children, grandchildren, and great-grandchildren.

Scriptural Reference:

> And the peace of God which passeth all understanding, shall keep your hearts and minds through Christ Jesus.

> Philippians 4:7

CHAPTER 13

▼

GRIEF AND LOSS

For this chapter I spoke to Vanessa A. Johnson, who lost both her mother and her son in a relatively short time. Vanessa has written a book entitled, *When Death Comes a Knockin'*. You can learn more about this author by visiting her web site at http://clik.to/vanessaajohnson. Please purchase a copy and read her entire story!

*   *   *   *

My mother, Arcadia "Grace" Alexander, was born on January 12, 1932. On Sunday August 28, 1994 during the early morning hours between one and two a.m., my mother had a massive heart attack while sitting on her bed staring out the window. As far as we knew, she had not had any other major health problems before then, certainly none that could have warned us prior to her attack.

My son Jalen Michael Johnson was born prematurely on February 17, 1994. Soon after learning I was pregnant with him, the doctors confirmed that he had a birth defect wherein his urethral valve was blocked. Throughout the pregnancy up until his birth, I went through surgical procedures to keep extracting the amniotic fluid from his abdomen and put it back into the amniotic sac. This problem caused him to be premature, and when I delivered at 32 weeks, he weighed 3 ½ pounds. He remained in the NICU (Neonatal Intensive Care Unit) for two months and was actually released the weekend he was to be born had the pregnancy gone to full term. After his release from the hospital he continued to thrive at home.

The only other time Jalen was hospitalized was on July 28, 1994 when he had to have intestinal mal-rotation surgery. But, he breezed through that and was released from the hospital on August 31, 1994. Then on September 19, 1994 he was admitted to the hospital for pneumonia. He seemed to be improving and was taken off of the ventilator on September 29. Obviously that proved too much for him, and he had difficulty breathing on his own. Early the following morning, September 30, he went into cardiac arrest, and well, the rest is history. The doctors said he must have aspirated on his baby food, but none of the tests they performed confirmed that theory. It was like he was doing fine one day, and the next he had pneumonia and was gone.

I'd be the first to tell you, I didn't handle those occurrences too well. As a matter of fact, everyday that passed after that, I sank deeper and deeper into depression—so much so that my husband became alarmed. It was after expressing his concern to a friend of his that the friend suggested I seek help through grief counseling. I knew I was in trouble, and I agreed to go because I knew that if I didn't, I might not make it myself. This truly was the lowest point of my life, but I knew I needed help, and I still had a 14-year old who was depending on me.

When I first joined grief counseling, I was distraught and angry. Oh so angry! I felt guilty that I, as Jalen's mother, couldn't do anything to save him. I felt guilty that I didn't insist they put him back on the ventilator when I saw him having difficulty breathing. I relied on the advice of the doctors when I should have relied on my instincts.

The grief counseling group helped me to sort out the feelings I was experiencing. Talking with other people who were going through the same things I was helped. I didn't feel so alone. I could talk to them if I wanted (which they encouraged). I could cry if I needed to without worrying about them tiring of hearing my sob story. And I learned to recognize the stages of the grief process—Disbelief, Anger, Bargaining, Depression, and Acceptance.

I attended grief counseling for a year. I stopped going because I felt like I was continuing to live in the past—that expressing my story and my feelings over and over again week after week was keeping me in the depression. I felt I was finally coming to terms with the loss of Mom and Jalen and was ready to move on. Do I still have my bad days when I revert back to stages (Anger and Depression) in the grief process? My answer is yes, I certainly do. In addition to grief counseling I started writing, and I used it as a tool to express what I was feeling, what I was going through in my grief. What started out as a seven-page essay has turned into a 146-page book which I've dedicated to my deceased loved ones. It's entitled *When Death Comes a Knockin'*. It is a self-help inspirational resource guide that details my experiences with loss and my journey through the grief process.

You know the old saying about life, *take one day at a time*. Well, I've learned that the saying for me was *take one second at a time*, because in a second your emotions can change, and you find yourself in an emotional whirlwind. Time has definitely played a part in my healing process. I go for longer periods of time before falling back into one of the stages of grief, and when I do fall back, my stay there is for shorter periods of time. Once you've lost a parent and a child, or any significant person in your life, I feel that you deal with your grief for a lifetime. I know that I will never forget my loved ones. I've just learned that I can keep them alive in my heart, and I can bring them out whenever I choose to and not fall apart.

*   *   *   *

Help Through Learning Other Persons' Stories

Sometimes anger will overwhelm the griever. Carole says that she was so mad at her cousin (who murdered Carole's mother) that she actually took a gun with her to the courtroom when she attended the trial. "Had the system refused to indict him, I was prepared to shoot him myself," Carole said.

Shortly after her mother's death, Carole sacrificed her career to care for her father, whom she watched die over an eleven-month period. Her dad suffered from renal failure, congestive heart failure, and emphysema.

Carole Weddington is a state licensed and nationally certified counselor, author, radio talk show host, consultant, and poet. She is the host of *GET A GRIP*, a phone coaching talk show on AdviceRadio.com. She has a graduate degree in Counseling from Delta State University and a B.A. in Psychology from the University of Mississippi. She continued her education at the University of Memphis and the University of Missouri at Columbia and completed 45 hours above her graduate degree. She is the founder of Creative Communications.

Carole has presented at national, regional, and state-wide conferences in the areas of anger management, traumatic grief, depression, substance abuse, relationships, women's issues, family violence, post-traumatic stress disorders, sexual abuse and ADHD. She has over 20 years of clinical experience from working with adolescent and adult psychiatric populations. She has developed programs for adolescent, adult psychiatric, and substance abuse in-patient and out-patient hospital programs. In addition she has supervised clinical teams in mental health settings prior to starting Creative Communications.

She is a member of the American Counseling Association, Association for Death Education and Counseling, and the American Association of Christian Counselors. She is also past president of the West Tennessee Counseling Association. Carole writes from her clinical and personal experiences. Personally she had to grieve the loss of her mother, who was brutally stabbed multiple times by her mother's nephew, and the death of her father. Beyond this trauma, she has endured a history of physical abuse from childhood to age 28 at the hands of her brother. She journeyed through grief and anger; then she was resurrected like a phoenix from the ashes.

Experience Carole's journey in D-ANGER I'M MAD! ANGER MANAGEMENT GOD'S STYLE, HELLO MR. D.: A JOURNEY THROUGH GRIEF and D+ANGER I'M MAD! ANGER MANAGEMENT TEEN STYLE. In addition, Carole has written two journal articles: "Sexual Abuse & ADHD" and "Grief & the Chemically Dependent." You can contact Carole at *CreativeCom1@aol.com.*

Scriptural Reference:

Hereafter shall the Son of man sit on the right hand of the power of God.

St. Luke 22:69

Resources

Most Frequently Asked Questions

The National Family Caregivers Association (NFCA) receives hundreds of phone calls and emails a week from family caregivers seeking resources, referrals and advice.

The following is a compilation of the most frequently asked questions (FAQs) and their responses.

1. **I'm looking for respite services. Whom should I contact?**

    NATIONAL ORGANIZATIONS AND PROGRAMS

    Easter Seals
    230 West Monroe Street, Suite 1800
    Chicago, IL 60606
    1-800-221-6827
    web: *www.easter-seals.org*
    email: *info@easter-seals.org*
    Provides a variety of services at 400 sites nationwide for children and adults with disabilities, including adult day care, in-home care, camps for special needs children and more. Services vary by site.

    <<<<<<]**Family Friends**
    National Council on the Aging, Inc.
    409 Third Street SW
    Washington, DC 20024
    202-479-6675 or 202-479-6672
    web: *www.ncoa.org*
    email: *miriam.charno@ncoa.org*

Provides respite for families of children with special needs by men and women volunteers over the age of 50. Programs located throughout the country—with 47 centers and over 2000 volunteers.
congregations working together. Services vary by site. There are currently 1300 programs throughout the country.

Shepherd's Centers of America
One West Armour Street, Suite 201
Kansas City, MO 64111
1-800-547-7073
web: *www.shepherdcenters.org*
email: *staff@shepherdcenters.org*
Provides respite care, telephone visitors, in-home visitors, nursing home visitors, home health aides, support groups, adult day care, and information and referrals for accessing other services available in the community. Services vary by center. There are currently 75 centers around the country.

REFERRAL SOURCES

National Association of Adult Day Services
National Council on the Aging
409 3rd Street SW, Suite 200
Washington, DC 20024
202-479-6682
web: *www.ncoa.org*
Provides information about locating adult day care centers in your local area

2. **Are there caregiver resources on the Internet?**

CAREGIVER WEBSITES

There are a variety of web sites that offer information and support for family caregivers. Many of these sites offer the ability to type in a zip code and obtain a list of local resources for home care, respite care, assisted living facilities, rehab facilities, hospice and other types of care. To locate other sites, type "FAMILY CAREGIVER" on any of the major search engines for a complete listing. Here are some of our favorites:

www.nfcacares.org
The home page of the National Family Caregivers Association. Explore this web site and find out more about caregiving, what NFCA has to offer, about projects and programs underway and those that are planned for the future.

www.caregiver.com
Internet home for Today's Caregiver Magazine. Site includes topic specific news-letters, online discussion lists, back issue articles, chat.

www.familycareamerica.com
Offers varied resources to meet caregivers' specific needs, in their own localities, provides caregiver support, solution sharing, and discussion forums.

ELDERCARE WEBSITES

There are a variety of websites that offer information and support about elder care. Type "ELDERCARE" on any of the major search engines for a comprehensive listing. Below are sites that we are familiar with and are good resources.

Each of the sites listed provides general geriatric health information, senior news and information, bulletin boards, etc. Many of these sites offer the ability to type in a zip code and obtain a list of local resources for home care, respite care, assisted living facilities, rehab facilities, hospice and other types of care.

www.caregiving.com
www.carescout.com
www.eldercorner.com
www.extendedcare.com

3. **Where can I find financial help for my caregiving?**

GENERAL RECOMMENDATIONS

Contact county or state Department of Health and Human Services or area social service agencies, such as Catholic Charities, Association of Jewish Family and Children's Agencies, and local chapters of voluntary health agencies to find out if they offer any financial support programs and how to apply for them.

PRESCRIPTION DRUG AND MEDICAL CARE SUPPORT PROGRAMS

Federal Hill-Burton Free Care Program
1-800-638-0742 (message center).
Offers referrals to agencies that offer free medical care.

Medicine Program
P.O. Box 520
Doniphan, MO 63935
1-573-996-7300
web: *www.themedicineprogram.com*
email: *help@themedicineprogram.com*
A means-tested program for persons who do not have coverage either through insurance or government subsidies for outpatient prescription drugs, and who cannot afford to purchase medications at retail prices.

Pharmaceutical Research and Manufacturers of America (PHRMA)
1100 Fifteenth Street, NW
Washington DC 20005
1-800-762-4636 (message center)
202-935-3400 to speak directly to someone
web: *www.phrma.org*
Provides a patient assistance directory that includes a list of pharmaceutical company-run programs to help people without insurance or those with a low income obtain medications

The Caregivers Marketplace
The Caregivers Group, Inc.
P.O. Box 1206
Charlestown RI 02813
Phone: 401-364-9100 Fax: 401-364-9933 Toll free: 1-866-327-8340
www.caregiversmarketplace.com
The Caregivers Marketplace™ offers discounts on the commonly used products for incontinence, nutrition, bathing, skin care, mobility, aids to daily living, and more.

4. **I'm looking for overall caregiver support. Where can I find it?**

GENERAL RECOMMENDATIONS

Contact your local hospital or clinic (social work department); county department of senior services or disability services, area adult day centers, social service agencies and/or the local chapter of the health agency that focuses on your loved one's condition. It is by no means certain that they will offer caregiver support services, but they are good places to check.

SPECIFIC ORGANIZATIONS

National Family Caregivers Association
10400 Connecticut Avenue Suite 500
Kensington, MD 20895
1-800-896-3650
web: *www.nfcacares.org*
email: *info@nfcacares.org*
The National Family Caregivers Association (NFCA) is a grassroots organization created to educate, support, empower and advocate for the millions of Americans who care for chronically ill, aged or disabled loved ones. NFCA is the only constituency organization that reaches across the boundaries of different diagnoses, different relationships and different life stages to address the common needs and concerns of all family caregivers. NFCA is the voice of family caregivers. Members receive the quarterly newsletter, Take Care!, inspirational greeting cards and access to an experienced staff which provides information, referrals and caregiver support counseling.

American Self-Help Clearinghouse
Northwest Covenant Medical Center
25 Pocono Road
Denville, NJ 07834
1-973-625-9565
web: *www.selfhelpgroups.org*
email: *ashc@cybernex.net*
Not caregiver specific, but serves as an information clearinghouse for self-help groups of all types and provides information on how to start a support group.

Family Caregiver Alliance (FCA) (in California only)
690 Market Street Suite 600
San Francisco, CA 94104
1-415-434-3388
1-800-445-8106 (CA only)
web: *www.caregiver.org*
email: *info@caregiver.org*
FCA is a nationally recognized information center on long-term care and the lead agency in California's system of Caregiver Resource Centers. FCA serves as a public voice for caregivers, illuminating the daily challenges they face, offering them the assistance they so desperately need and deserve, and championing their cause through education, services, research and advocacy.

Friends Health Connection
PO Box 114
New Brunswick, NJ 08903
800-384-7436
web: *www.48friend.org*
email: *FHC@pilot.NJIN.NET*
Links persons with illness or disability and their family caregivers with others experiencing the same challenges.

Well Spouse Foundation
30 East 40th Street PH
New York, NY 10016
1-800-838-0879
web: *www.wellspouse.org*
A national, not for profit membership organization which gives support to husbands, wives and partners of the chronically ill and/or disabled. They offer support group information for spouses.

5. **Where can I find information about caring for my aging parents and related family issues?**

    GENERAL RECOMMENDATIONS

    Contact your county department of senior services or elder affairs, area adult day centers, and/or social service agencies providing services to the elderly.

    REFERRAL SOURCES

    AARP
    601 E Street, NW
    Washington, DC 20049
    1-800-424-3410
    web: *www.aarp.org*
    Supplies education and information about caregiving, long-term care, and aging, including publications and audio-visual aids for caregivers.

    Children of Aging Parents (CAPS)
    1609 Woodbourne Road #302A
    Levittown, PA 19057
    1-800-227-7294
    www.experts.com
    www.careguide.net

CAPS assists caregivers of the elderly with information and referrals, a network of support groups, and publications and programs that promote public awareness of the value and the needs of caregivers.

Eldercare Locator
National Association of Area Agencies on Aging
927 15th Street, NW 6th floor
Washington, DC 20005
1-800-677-1116
web: *www.n4a.org.*
Referrals to Area Agencies on Aging via zip code locations. Offers information about many eldercare issues and services in local communities.

The National Association of Professional Geriatric Care Managers
1604 North Country Club Road
Tucson, AZ 85716
1-520-881-8008
web: *www.caremanager.org*
Geriatric care managers (GCMs) are health care professionals, most often social workers, who help families in dealing with the problems and challenges associated with caring for the elderly. This national organization will refer you to their state chapters, which in turn can give you the names of GCMs in your area.

6. **How do I go about locating home care help or an assisted living or nursing facility?**

WATCHDOG ORGANIZATIONS

Consumer Consortium on Assisted Living
PO Box 3375
Arlington, VA 22203
1-703-841-2333
CCAL is a national consumer-focused organization that is dedicated to representing the needs of residents in assisted living facilities and educating consumers, professionals, and the general public about assisted living issues. Authored the book "Choosing an Assisted Living Facility, Strategies for Making the Right Decision" which provides helpful information and contains a concise questionnaire.

National Citizens Coalition for Nursing Home Reform
1424 Sixteenth Street, NW Suite 202

Washington, DC 20036
1-202-332-2275
web: *www.nccnhr.org*
email: *nccnhr@nccnhr.org*
Serves as an information clearinghouse; offers referrals nationwide for help with concerns about long-term care facilities.

REFERRAL SOURCES

Senior Alternatives
1-800-350-0770
web: *www.senioralternatives.com*
Publishes regional directories of nursing homes, assisted living and retirement communities. Call for a free copy or visit them on the web.

Visiting Nurses Association of America
11 Beacon Street Suite 910
Boston, MA 02108
617-523-4042
web: *www.vnaa.org*
email: *vnaa@vnaa.org*
Promotes community based home health care. You can contact them to find your local VNA.

7. **How do I find training to improve my caregiving skills, and how do I learn skills to help me cope better with the stresses of caregiving?**

GENERAL RECOMMENDATIONS

Community-based organizations periodically offer classes and workshops for family caregivers. Check your local paper for listings. Also check with your local community college, hospital or Red Cross chapter, and the local chapter of the voluntary health agency focused on your loved one's illness or disability.

Strength for Caring
1-888-422-7380
web: *www.oncolink.upenn.edu/sfc*
A national program to train cancer caregivers does exist.

Web Sites About Loss and Grief
www.grieflossrecovery.com

www.geocities.com/griefhope
www.compassionconnection.org
www.compassionatefriends.org
www.bereavedfamilies.net
www.beyondindigo.com
www.goodgrief.org
www.rivendell.org (GriefNet.Org)
http://my.freeway.net/~poetman
www.griefhealing.com
www.groww.com
www.journeyofhearts.org
www.thecomfortofhome.com
www.selfhealingexpressions.com
www.rfgifts.com

ELDERCARE NOTES

Name

Address

Phone

Nearest Intersection

MEDICATIONS

Daily

With Meals

Bedtime

IN AN EMERGENCY

Call 911 or: Phone

Doctor   Phone

Family Member   Daytime phone
                        Evening phone
Family Member   Daytime phone
                        Evening phone
Neighbor   Phone

ADDITIONAL INFORMATION

Medication Record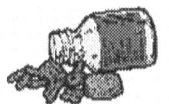

Name _____

Physician's Name _____

Physician's Address _____

Physician's Phone Number _____

Pharmacy Name _____

Pharmacy Phone Number_____

Keep the following list with you at all times:

Date Medication Started_____ / _____ / _____
Name of Medication _____
Dosage _____

Date Medication Started_____ / _____ / _____
Name of Medication _____
Dosage _____

Date Medication Started_____ / _____ / _____
Name of Medication _____
Dosage _____

Date Medication Started_____ / _____ / _____
Name of Medication _____
Dosage _____

Date Medication Started_____ / _____ / _____
Name of Medication _____
Dosage _____

Date Medication Started_____ / _____ / _____
Name of Medication _____
Dosage _____

Caregiver Daily Prayer Journal

DATE

Caregiver Daily Prayer Journal

DATE

Caregiver Daily Prayer Journal

DATE

Caregiver Daily Prayer Journal

_____ DATE _____

Caregiver Daily Prayer Journal

DATE _____

_____

_____

_____

_____

_____

_____

_____

_____

_____

_____

_____

_____

_____

_____

_____

_____

_____

_____

_____

_____

Caregiver Daily Prayer Journal

DATE

Caregiver Daily Prayer Journal

DATE

Outline of Home-going Ceremony

Processional...............
Prayer...............
Scripture...............
Solo...............
Acknowledgments...............
Obituary...............Read by...............or Read Silently
Solo...............
Remarks...............
Words of Comfort...............(Minister)
Review...............(Solo)...............
Benediction
Recessional
Committal and Interment...............

Appreciation

The family wishes to acknowledge with deep appreciation the many comforting messages, prayers, and many other expressions of kindness. You will receive a more formal thank you at a later time. May God richly bless you.

Pallbearers

Honorary Pallbearers

Flower Bearers

About the Author

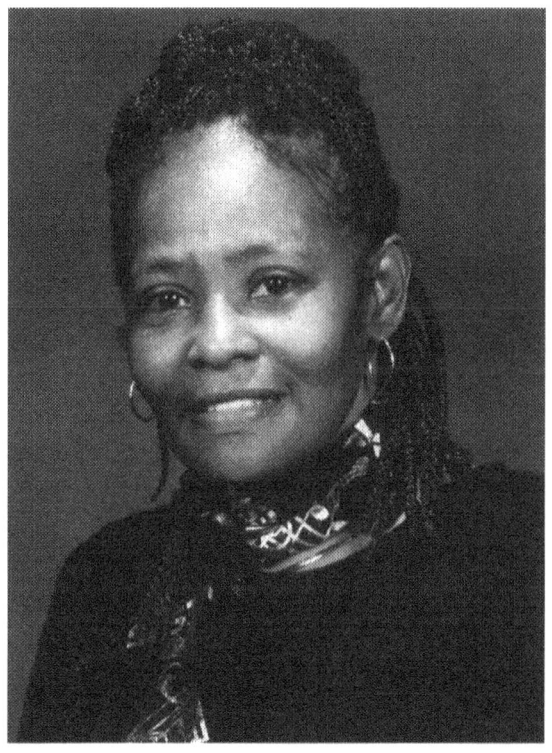

Delores Thornton

Delores Thornton, a lifelong Indianapolis resident, belongs to several writing organizations including her own Marguerite Press (www.margueritepress.com), founded in 1996; Marguerite Press Promo, founded in 2003; and Black Writers On Tour. She is the host of "A Round 2 It," an Internet radio show on www.deloresthornton.com. Thornton is a columnist for the *Indiana Herald* newspaper and for *The HYPE Magazine.* Additionally she is the literary expert on www.blackrefer.com and writes a monthly column at www.doenetwork.com, "How To Self-publish That Great Novel Without Going Nuts!" She freelances for Oneswan Productions, an Internet site. There are also links to her works found at www.cbbooksdistribution.com.

Thornton started writing in 1995, and friends encouraged her to publish her first novel, *Ida Mae*, in 1997. Her second work, *Ida Mae: The Saga Continues*, was released in 1998. In May 2000, she released *Ida Mae* as a combined edition. Her third novel, *Babe* was released in December 2000. *Anybody Seen Junebug?*, voted "Book of the Year 2003" by Disilgold Publishing, was published by iUniverse in 2003.

In March of 2001 Thornton and her novels were featured in a 30 minute video by the United States Postal Service. Filmed at the Mail Processing Annex in Indianapolis, the video was shown in postal installations worldwide. Thornton, a retired postal worker, contributed regularly to the "Postal Newsletter" in Indianapolis. In 2003 she wrote the highlights of the *Black Ourstory* celebration, which she coordinated for Black History Month. She also covered the *Employee Appreciation Day* held in June 2003.

The sought-after Thornton does motivational speaking and gives workshops and seminars. Favorite topics of facilitation include "Divine Intentions," "Seven Steps to Success (or 7 Sweet Ps)," "Self-publishing," and "Small Business Start-up."

In 1999, Thornton was approached by Audra Snyder Bailey, a ninety-year-old retired Indiana schoolteacher-turned-author who was in need of a distributor. A few years earlier Bailey had penned a book, *Hold Fast To Dreams,* and was dissatisfied with her contract. Thornton created new contracts and began to represent her, taking Bailey's books along with her own. In 2000 Bailey wrote a chapter about Thornton in her release *Heartbeat of the Heartland: People You'll Be Glad to Know.*

In addition to countless signings at bookstores and libraries, Thornton has addressed students at South High School in Columbus, Ohio; a Girl Scout troop at University United Methodist Church, Indianapolis; classes at Indiana University and also Martin University where her novels have been part of its convocation programs; middle-school students in Beaumont, Texas; the "Celebration of African-American Womanhood," South Bend, Indiana; attendees aboard the "First African-American Book Club Summit at Sea, Cancun, Mexico; the Baltimore Book Festival 1999 and 2001; Words Escape Me Summit, Birmingham, Alabama; Visions and Words, Oakland, California; and Writers & Poets 2001,

Detroit, Michigan. Thornton has also been featured in online chats hosted by Destee of Destee.com, Heather Covington at Disilgold.com, and Thumper at AALBC.com.

Thornton has traveled extensively promoting her work and has gained a loyal readership. She has been awarded certificates from Journey's End Literary Club and Sistah Circle Book Club. In 2000 her debut novel *Ida Mae* won the "Black Book of the Year" award from UBUS (United Brothers and United Sisters) of Richmond, Virginia. She was recognized at "Meet the Artists XIII" by the Indianapolis Marion County Public Library. Her novel *Babe* won "Best Book of 2002" on the Book Crazy Listener Awards.

Thornton has been featured in *The Michigan Bulletin*, *The Washington Post*, *The Sacramento Bee*, *Scoop*, *The Black Voice*, *Newsletter of the Black Caucus of the American Library Association*, *The Indianapolis Star*, *The Indianapolis Recorder*, and *Indiana Herald*.

On July 4, 2002, Thornton launched her *Around 2 It* radio show on 1310 AM in Indianapolis. The format provided a forum for authors, singers, poets, and other artists. Operating under the parent company, Marguerite Press, the show sponsored an essay contest which awarded trophies and other prizes to children in grades two through twelve. In December of 2002 the *Around 2 It* radio talk show moved to the Internet.

Thornton helped her friend Lena Williams launch the "Friend Gurlz Book Club" in 2002. The club has participated in community service work and is bringing authors to the Indianapolis area.

Voted the "Literary Queen/2003" by C&B Books Distribution of New York, Thornton has tried to share her knowledge with others. To that end she brought authors together under the umbrella of her Marguerite Press Yahoo Group. The email group is free to join and members are privy to tons of information!

After advertising in mainstream catalogs and paying hundreds of dollars, Thornton felt that she could design one at a comparable price. She began offering souvenir books for her literary functions, and they were so enthusiastically received that she decided to branch out and offer author catalogs. Always one with novel ideas, Thornton has a contract with a local band in Indianapolis, Exact Change, whose members record companion CDs for her work. This has proven to be an outstanding marketing tool, and now the music is available at *www.CDBaby.net*. The band promotes the books as they perform at area nightclubs and other venues. Thornton has designed and sold T-shirts, ink pens, front license plates, calendars, and tote bags.

Thornton also holds an annual "Small Press Awards" program. Entrants submit a business profile, and people are invited to send an email vote for the candidate of their choice. In 2003 the awards will also acknowledge the "Best Author Site," "Best Publicist," and "Best Promoter."

In July of 2003 the ever-busy Thornton was asked to judge an online beauty pageant and a self-published book awards program!

Thornton is a graduate of Indiana Business College and the LongRidge Writers Group of West Redding, CT. She has taken board governance and non-profit organization courses at the Indianapolis Neighborhood Resource Center. A literacy volunteer with Indy Reads, Thornton attends Simmons Bible College in Indianapolis, and is currently working on her next title, *Family Matters: Airing Dirty Linen,* due out in 2005. When she has spare time, Thornton enjoys long drives and visiting with her grown children and grandchildren.

Delores Thornton is available for speaking engagements, seminars, and workshops. Contact her at: *dthorn4047@aol.com.* Phone: (317) 626-6885.

Airing Dirty Linen

by Delores Thornton. Release date 2005.

To the casual observer it might have appeared that the Dobson family had healed with a suddenness. In actuality that couldn't have been further from the truth. The four cousins had seen their share of misery and had been the subject of all types of investigations. When their parents died, they inherited loads of money and invested it wisely—in a lavish bed and breakfast on picturesque Allisonville Place. Yet the problems didn't end. The bed and breakfast had plenty of walk-in closets, each with it's own share of skeletons. But, they were a private group, and private things rarely got out.

0-595-31897-5